MAKE

WORLDS

Doctor Jean-François Huber

Birth of a Neuromedicine

Translated from French by Dr. William John Stuart

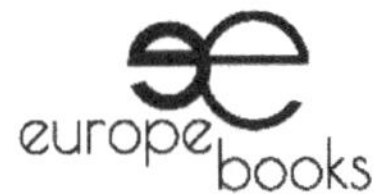

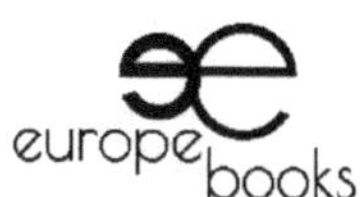

Birth of a Neuromedicine

Dedicated to Julien, Pierre, and Nicole, To Raymonde, Isabelle, Olivier and Cécile, and also Mathilde, Paul-Henri, Justine, Louis, Romane, Eliot, Oscar, and Jean.

This book is dedicated to them, as it is to them I owe all my desire to live.

Preface

I am a rural general practitioner, and I have discovered neuromedicine.

I can imagine a skeptical response to this proposition in a world of medicine where the roads to a cure seem already established and that for about 2 centuries by research doctors and their various followers. However...

I made this discovery in the early days of my practice of medicine, and I have never since stopped finding support for my theories. For over 30 years of my practicing neuromedicine their validity is quite apparent.

My approach is both an innovation and rooted in the history of medicine from the ancient practitioners. It assigns to the nervous system a rule of thumb that has not yet been allowed to it in current medical thought. I am not discussing the mind here, but the neurological functions of our bodies, the so-called "Black Box" of Jean Pierre Changeux. (1) The nervous system is a tripartite one that consists of body functions such as organ functions, motricity and sensibility; brain functioning or mind operations in the neocortex; and energy management in the paleocortex, the fight and flight reactions to stress, and in the archeocortex, where adaptation occurs, which is essential for life.

This nervous unit, where energy is managed, should become the focus of a new medicine in order to redefine the criteria for future medical care. For it is involved in all our current diseases.

Only the techniques of re-education through simulating nerve endings allow effective treatment for these functional neurological disorders from which diseases arise.

The concept of medical therapy must now take into consideration the neuroscientific aspect of each disease and treatment must reflect this. We can no longer merely passively treat diseases with drugs.

Neuromedicine is anchored in an examination of the sensibility of the cutaneous tissues.

Its examination is an undeniable diagnostic and follow-up tool. It reveals recent or past unconscious neurological events, whether physical or psychological in origin.

My personal history as a practitioner will provide readers with the keys to understand how neuromedicine got started. Much influenced by my early medical school knowledge and early mastery of mesotherapy techniques, hydrological techniques used in thermal baths, I developed neuromedicine over the years while diagnosing and treating thousands of patients often with neglected chronic diseases i.e. unresponsive to other treatments.

I took interest in numerous minor diseases causing pain, making the patient's life miserable. Early detection and treatment prevented chronicity and exacerbation from occurring, which would certainly have evolved without intervention.

Neuromedicine derives from an ineluctable adage: the patients hold the key to their own cure. Thus I chose to apply this non-specific type of re-educative rehabilitating treatment that does not directly involve muscles, organ functions, or mental functions. The patient's betterment is obtained through local neurostimulation whereby one elicits an improvement through adaptation and energetic global recovery.

Neuromedicine is neither an alternative medicine falling into the category of any type of medicine that does not use drugs nor is it a therapeutic technique. It is an all-encompassing holistic approach but with definite limitations. There are precise indications making it an unavoidable alternate choice.

More than merely getting promising results, I have described a scientific procedure that comprises methods, goals and indications.

I am well aware of its limitations: they have more to do with the severity of a disease than its nature.

One needs to be a perspicacious observer and clinician to be a doctor. But it also takes an all-encompassing vision, it takes confidence in the ability of a patient to get well, it takes trust in the life force humankind has. This is always expressed more as a certainty of a better future than as the regrets of a painful past.

To give care, to cure is a break with the past, but it is also the start of a hopeful future.

There always arises the question of "How does it work?"

It is often asked from a negative bias before even accepting that it works. To standardize the results and be able to compare them to similar patients, one has to agree on the mode of action. What is in common with acute and chronic diseases, old and young, between conventional medicine and the reductive medicine of neurostimulation?

Doesn't it come to mind to anyone that the current medical methodology is just a step in the evolution of medical practices from those initial beginnings? Not to say that certain principles of conventional medicine are not excellent, they are. Moreover, results are well-founded, and the competence of the caregivers very good.

That which is transitory is the dogma and the single-minded thinking. In order to be in line with the theories of conventional medicine I speak without any problem of placebo-effect in this book. For the indications where my technique works, there are from 20-50 % good results. In re-educative neurostimulation there is inevitably a good result to some extent.

I am aware of the questions this type of medicine might generate. An evident contradiction exists between the intention to give a patient his autonomy and applying conventional techniques which prevent him for the most part from being his own referee. There is also an incongruity between how the patient demands a good quality of life, but gives little significance to their health picture. Through neurostimulation, one gives back to the patient their capacity to adapt, to be in control of their life.

In the history of medicine from the very start, certain physicians have sounded an alarm to bring doctors back to a patient's bedside. I espouse to be one of those physicians. Doctors, but also patients, must be re-educated to see disease in another light and even redefine the notion of health.

I am currently preparing another book, which will be a manual for the Practice of neuromedicine for Medical Practitioners and other health professionals. It will contain a guide to rolling palpation and a description of how to carry out the treatment of multiple subcutaneous microinjections using the various products which compose the drugs used. Both the techniques of injecting and the specifications of drugs will be explained.

I will also be available to hold training sessions in my medical center for interested parties that respond to the book.

This book is addressed to the general public, to my peers, and especially to my patients. It is adressed to those who for so long, through their confidence, allowed me to build this new, unique medical science. It is a step closer to patients solving their problems as chief actors in their health.

The ultimate goal is not to cure a disease but to stimulate the patient to heal themselves.

1 You will be a doctor

"This is the medicine of my life. I understood that patients hold the key to their own cure."

A great family

My paternal Grandfather, son of a physician in Amiens, was a pediatrician and Professor at the School of Medicine in Paris. His wife was a rich bourgeois heiress, although a rural one, whose family got rich through a rock quarry business near Mantes-la-Jolie. This family became wealthy in furnishing the foundation blocks of the Arc de Triumph. From about 1890 to 1900, my great grandfather used to hunt in and around Vetheuil, Mantes-la-Jolie, La Roche-Guyon and also Chérence, where he lived. Legend has it that he crossed paths with Claude Monet on occasion. What's more, it seems that they both had an affair with the same woman...

My maternal relatives were "Lords of the Land" or longstanding farmers, nobles not in the spotlight, but very attached to the land and its history. The role of each generation was to perpetuate, through passed on knowledge, a farming profession lasting 600 years...

My future was programmed for me. However, I resisted it for a while. I said to myself, "If I want, I won't go there. I can study law or become a priest. And why not a farmer?" I liked Nature, which always has inspired me. As a young man, I dreamed of all the doors open to me. Most of all, I was not going to subject myself to bow to the Establishment. I was different, a proud individual, and I had no concern about having a bright future or not.

A profession

I took my time with my High School Diploma in hand to finally get admitted to the Montpellier School of Medicine. I was a loner, thinking all the time, and my personality wasn't very compatible with the usual university studies. I advanced with difficulty among academic structures, which were much too rigid for me. Then two major events occurred. I got married, and we had a child. I had no doubt about my choice, and I was very happy. These events opened for me a double role, that of student and head of a family, at 23 years old. I soon found work in a hospital as night nurse, of course. Everything interested me. I knew I would be a General Practitioner, a specialist in general medicine. I wanted to study the heart, the lungs, the gut, but most of all, be close to my patients.

I was drawn to these fragile patients and the lack of stability put on display by their poor health. I was under the impression I was here to restore their autonomy. I wanted to give them back who they were. "We are going to repair it, but it's up to you. It does not belong to me, but to you."

One day, at the Montpellier Hospital Psychiatric ward, they gave me a young boy to examine, a known violent psychotic patient. I found myself alone with him. My group of students stood behind a one-way mirror and watched us. At the end of the 20 minutes, when the session was over, the Resident Doctor in charge of my group asked me, "How did you do that?"

I already had the talent to speak gently but firmly, to approach a patient without fear.

It was a fact that in the puritan conception of the world which I had, disease bothered me. I felt like I had to find a reason for the disease. There was little chance I would adhere to the official doctrines... Trained by my mother to make new out of old, I became a recycle doctor. Bring me your disease, we will make something new out of it.

I worked in the hospital as nurse, house officer, and resident. In 1974, I was the night nurse for the first kidney transplant recipients... But it was really in 1976 in Palavas where my true medical adventure began.

First as a nurse, then as a resident doctor, I was employed to assist in the surgical operations of Professor Jean Gabriel Pous, who had established a Department of Pediatric Surgery with Professor Alain Dimeglio and his team in Montpellier. They carried out correctional procedures on children with clubfoot, congenital hip dysplasia, spinal paralysis, Pott's Disease. Using orthopedic techniques, they extended or shortened lower limbs in children affected by poliomyelitis. They cut the long bone in two so that bone would form at the extremities little by little, all the while increasing the distance between proximal and distal parts each day. It was High Tech medicine and really fascinating.

In this Department, I learned to examine the shoulders, hips, the spine, and take care of scoliosis. This experience was very useful to me.

Roscoff, or the revelation

In 1979 I left Palavas to take up a job at The Institute of Marine Therapy, run by Dr. René Bagot at Roscoff in North Britany on the coast. My main motivation for taking this job was purely pecuniary. I had of course all the disdain you could expect from a medical scholar for this kind of medicine.

Dr. Bagot treated about 3,500 patients over a six-month period of time. There were three young doctors (including me) doing intake procedures, filling out initial records in order that a daily journal could be made. The first 2 months were rough going, and I thought I wouldn't stay on much more. But then I had a flash of inspiration. I saw the light of neurologic re-education: A revelation. The word is strong, especially for me, who showed little enthusiasm. I now realised that patients themselves held the key to their own cure.
I found the medicine of my life.

Hydrotherapy and sea water therapy. It was Roscoff! A completely new world for me. It was here that all got started. It was in Roscoff that the rolling palpation technique and reflex massage techniques were engraved in my memory. It was here that Louison Bobet, three time Tour de France winner, was trained. As an anecdote, when he created his first center in Quiberon, he took with him many doctors working at Dr. Bagot's Center. Bobet discovered the capability of sea water therapy to improve pain and especially the phenomenal utility of the rolling palpation technique. Phenomenal because it is certainly surprising to find traces of a patient's suffering and even his past clinical history inscribed in their skin.

Thanks to my training at Palavas I had learned well how to examine the bones and joints. There was only left for me to be vigilant about the contraindications of thermal baths. I saw 15-20 patients per day in this setting which promotes rehabilitation of a patient more than directly treating his disease. In sea water therapy, as in thermal bath cures, we were not dealing with acute illnesses but chronic ones. Patients had been in pain for a long time. I cared for them and tried to alleviate their pains. I could feel that what I treated was undoubtedly a mixture of disease and sheer unhappiness: a condensation of pathology and life experience.

Dr. Bagot was not a psychologist, but he was pragmatic. He showed me other new perspectives. When a patient failed to respond and still complained of sharp pains, he got out a syringe from his pocket, filled it with a diluted solution of xylocaine (an anesthetic) and injected it locally as an intradermal where the pain existed according to the rolling palpation technique. This way he created a very superficial papula. The objective of his technique was not to inject a painkiller in the site of pain. Behind his jabs, something else was at play; they provoked a reaction that brought the patient out from the shackles of their disease.

I hoped to stay on at Roscoff. I could see myself as eventually taking over for Dr. Bagot. But this didn't happen. I began working as resident doctor in Bagnols Sur Ceze General Hospital in the Gard in the South of France. I sure didn't appreciate this return to the South of France. Brittany, secular and beautiful, clean with its disciplined and determined population, had impressed me. And in the back of my mind I felt that maybe in leaving sea water therapy I was abandoning a career which could have been a brilliant one, founded upon an innovative medicine inspired by pioneers. Bagot was Patton... who kicked out conventional medicine and its one-way outlook. In his stead, I could have spread the word of sea water therapy worldwide, but this dream was shattered.

Return to traditional medicine

I took up a position in Cardiology, where I renewed the medical practices of my initial beginnings. I remained resident for several years, because, as head of the family, I was more interested in earning money than in completing my thesis. I eventually finished it in 1981 on "Genetics in Orthopedics", a subject given to me by Professor Alain Dimeglio. I was finally officially a Medicinae Doctor. From the time I started at the hospital I told a surgeon friend of mine, "If you have any sciatic patients send them over to me as I am interested in treating them..."

In reality, I had never jabbed an acute sciatic patient, but, strongly believing in my rolling palpation technique, I understood what should be done. In this fashion I soon treated about a dozen patients per week. Although never having had a particular training in mesotherapy techniques, I developed my own personal variant of it. I used jabs exclusively, with a diluted solution of xylocaine which I had discovered at Roscoff.

Later I did a locum tenens in Lapalud not far from Avignon. Already, I couldn't give up on using these jabs. As soon as I had examined a patient and the diagnosis gave me the possibility to help this person, I would not hesitate: I jabbed. This permitted me to establish appropriate diagnoses, such as in the young rugby player who said he had stomachache. With the rolling palpation technique, I could tell he had a small fracture of a thoracic vertebra in T7 or T8.

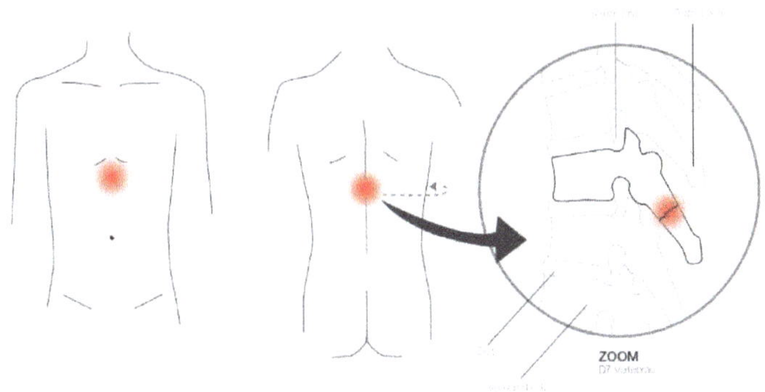

Word of mouth was effective and patients came in great numbers to see me. When the local doctor returned, he remarked, a bit frustrated, "But what did you do to them?" I hit the mark.

I did another locum tenens at Laudun L'Ardoise in the Gard for Dr. Diego Rodriguez and got the same response. When he returned, he said surprisingly, "It is good what you do. I don't understand it, but you seem to really help these patients." Later he asked me to become his General Practitioner partner, and eventually I did. When his wife saw the Waiting Room, full to the brim on Market Day in the afternoon, she exclaimed with surprise, "But this is Lourdes!"

In 1985, I met a mesotherapist who was looking to create a surgery devoted strictly to mesotherapy. But from the start of our discussions he made an interesting remark: "Listen, Huber, I want to do mesotherapy. "...but Huber-otherapy is out of the question."

A sign that neuromedecine had been taking shape for a long time now. He understood that, but not me, not just yet.

My colleague understood that I brought to light a system that he didn't believe in and didn't want to be a part of. He had learned to do jabs with mesotherapy drugs and was not about to do anything else. It was in vain that I tried to convince him that my work was a neurological form of re-eduction. I wanted to convince him at all costs because I was not going to change. Otherwise, I would have been in a contradiction of life and reality. As he would not let go of what he thought to be real and since we had different opinions on the matter, our common project never got off the ground.

Now, this is where an important turning point occurred defining neuromedicine: I had an intuition about it, but no proof. I completed this first series which consisted of treating patients with local intradermic injections of diluted xylocaine solution. I learned that xylocaine relieved pain in a first instance, like a drug, but over time it acted more like a re-educative stimulant. I discovered later that with Iodugluthional, an old drug derived from iodine and sulphur used in mesotherapy, not an anesthetic, the results were the same on Day 2. These jabs were capable of stimulating the body to bring it to grips with the causal disease. It is this neurostimulation that makes re-educative medicine so valuable. It is essential to make these patients come out of their usual neurologic framework and to bring them by this transitory aggravation to form a new balance which results in a cure.

It is essential to make these patients come out of their usual neurologic framework and to bring them by this transitory aggravation to form a new balance which results in a cure.

I now had the methodology but not the theoretical basis.

This is an important difference.

Creation of a medical theory

Very soon, I wanted to back up my results with medical concepts. From 1985 on I began to describe these concepts thanks to my daily discoveries. A systematisation of my diagnoses and treatment was developed. Ten to fifteen years were needed to describe the special map of dermatomes – we will discuss this later – and then another ten to fifteen years to complete my work of describing re-education with a holistic approach to the patient. I was influenced in this by numerous authors. One of them comes to mind, Jean Bossy, Professor of Neurology at the University of Montpellier, who wrote profusely on acupuncture.

The more I advanced in my thinking, the more I realised that neuromedicine was unique as a neuroscience as compared to classical medical sciences. Each patient brought wheat to my grist mill, reinforcing the cohesiveness of my theories and supporting my initial intuitions: I stimulated the neurologic system as a whole, as an actor in health, not as an individual organ.

But I was alone in this evolution of neuromedicine. It was difficult, since I was a remote rural doctor and because I was particularly busy with the economic success of my own medical practice.

Nevertheless, I felt the need to exchange opinions, to communicate with colleagues. My practice derived from mesotherapeutical techniques that were inspired by Dr. Pistor, so logically I associated with mesotherapists.

2 Mesotherapy, yes but...

"A little for Pistor and a little against Pistor, but always 'with' Pistor."

Some background history: Dr. Pistor

Michel Pistor, General Practitioner at Bray-et-Lû in the Val-d'Oise Department 60 km from Paris, went to the school of René Leriche, well known medical philosopher, and Lyon Surgeon between the Great Wars. He had worked on pain and in particular that related to the sympathetic nervous system.

René Leriche treated myocardial infection with infiltrations at the stellar ganglion, located at the summit of the lungs. If the patient did not die immediately from the shock of the procaïne injection, or of a pneumo thorax due to needle penetration of the pleura, then the stellar infiltration had a good chance of relieving the pain of the person whose vital prognosis was in play. At the time, the outcome of a myocardioal infarction was nearly always fatal.

Professor Leriche treated lots of patients with injections of procaine in the nerve plexus notably for the treatment of algodystrophy.

These reflex pain pathologies of the orthosympathetic nervous system resulted in trophic problems in the limb which was affected often, including muscle wasting. They sometimes were caused by the simple prick of a rose thorn!

Dr. Bagot of Roscoff often referred to Pr Leriche. Despite the different medical lines of thought, we are all derived from the same family, we are offspring of René Leriche!

In 1952 in line with Pr Leriche, Dr. Pistor, injected procaine into the neck of a shoemaker of Bray-et-Lû to treat wry neck. This patient returned to see him the next day and explained that just after the injection behind the ear, he had heard the sound of the village church bells, which he hadn't heard for twenty years. And rightly so for he was totally deaf. Dr. Pistor gave him another injection right away, but the shoemaker never did hear the bells again.

No miracle cure.

Dr. Pistor invented mesotherapy in this period. He continued to treat his patients with local injections of procaïne with which he added certain drugs, benefitting from the arrival of them in the 60s. With his technique, he treated everything, even presbytery, with small injections around the eyes. The drugs he usually used were from before the War: lodugluthional, peridil-heparine (a relatively strong vasodilator), divasta (an antistaphylococcic vaccine with surprising local and general reactions). It is of importance to remark that mesotherapy for a long time used drugs whose specificity was far from well-established. These drugs later disappeared from use.

Michel Pistor left Bray-et-Lû at the beginning of the 60s to establish himself in Paris. He founded the French Mesotherapy Society. He surrounded himself with a team among whom there was Dr. Bicheron. These illustrious pioneers had ideas about everything and treated all pathologies. Their treatments were often successful, in a time when medicine didn't have the means we possess nowadays.

Dr. Michel Pistor built a good reputation. He became recognised as an authority in many medical circles who invited him for presentations. His medical prowess exceeded the borders of France and was established in numerous countries.

In the 60s the modern medical dogma of conventional medicine was not yet established.

It was the stage of learning how to use new drugs such as antibiotics or cortisone. There was a lot left to discover.

Professors of medicine were still open-minded. In line with the wandering around that medicine was caught up in, it was admitted that even though there was a lot they could not explain, some of it could be real. Efficiency and results were respected. And mesotherapy worked.

Despite the fact that my grandfather had finished his hospital career, in 1965 he was Honorary President of the French Mesotherapy Society. He was a member of the National Academy of Medicine where he allowed Dr. Pistor to make the first presentation of mesotherapy.

So mesotherapy developed in parallel with conventional medicine. New and efficient in its beginnings, it suffered the consequences of the brilliant successes of conventional medicine, which was organised like a war machine ever since the creation of the Teaching Hospitals by Rober t Debré in 1962. Today there is no contest. Its: mesotherapy = 2, conventional medicine = 98. I don't mean to downtrod the revolution of conventional medicine. In many cases, it made unheard-of advances in medicine and developed our critical thinking. But for all that, I consider that it shouldn't presume such a complete hegemony. Dogma is a contradiction to the scientific method to which it adheres to with such authority. It is brilliant in treating more stable patients than in those recurrent benign cases and chronic diseases. In these indications, the results are limited and so transitory. It is efficient in reaching a cure, but lays aside prevention. It favors in the long term the emergence of chronic conditions with a risk of decompensation into a severe pathology. Putting sophisticated drugs on the market all the time also caused a big deficit in the health care system budget.

Today the French Mesotherapy Society is one of the most prosperous groups of scholarly doctors. There are about 800 members. Mesotherapy is used in about 30 countries. If it can leave some preset ideas behind, as we shall see, by combining efficient treatment and prevention, it has the potential to be a brilliant medicine for the future.

Pistor and I

In 1950, my parents lived in Chérence a small town of the Val d'Oise located on top of the limestone cliffs that dominate the Seine River between Vétheuil and la Roche-Guyon. So when I was one and a half years and had a pilonidal cyst, it was Dr. Pistor who treated me at Bray-et-Lû. He was our family doctor. He operated on this abscess and I still have a nasty scar. I made him laugh many years afterwards when I told him he probably inoculated me with the mesotherapy virus.

At the beginning of my academic career, I must admit I held him and his followers in low esteem. Like doctors do when just finished with medical school. To me he was... an acupuncturist at best. Even my father criticised him. When he wished to consult over joint pains, he asked if he should bring his x-ray films. Dr. Pistor said it would not be necessary. My father never again went to see him. A Doctor who consulted without using x-ray films was obviously a charlatan...

I knew he existed, that he treated arthritic pain and that he had good results. I was aware of the microinjections he used. I didn't think much of it until my revelation in seawater therapy with Dr. Bagot on Roscof f who used these same intradermal injections. This led me to the very personalised practice of a form of mesotherapy.

Dr. Pistor was with me throughout my life. Sometimes I was for Pistor, sometimes against him, but always with him.

When I met him for the first time at the mesotherapy convention at Balaruc Les Bains near Montpellier, he recognised me as the grandson of my grandfather, nothing more.

In another congress at Toulouse in 1996, I gave him an article I wrote entitled: "The Future of Mesotherapy: Microdose Conventional Medicine or Neurological Re-education?"

I saw him pass the paper to the current president and then... nothing happened.

Michel Pistor would probably have had the ability to open up to me, but by then, he was too old to do so. He was too old to take part in the re-positioning for power that was raging inside this scholarly society at that time.

I was happy to have known him. He was an authority to me for a long time, but his influence decreased over the years through the brief relations we had in the years before his passing in 2003.

Mesotherapy: a definition

According to Pistor, mesotherapy is defined as a form of conventional medicine using micro dosages of drugs. Thus very little drug and rarely. It is recognised as effective for pain relief and is branching out into cosmetic medicine. Through clinical examination and thorough questioning, the mesotherapist reveals the patient's zones of suffering that often relate to underlying pathologies.

Then he injects into the skin in small doses drugs that correspond to the specific pathology.

Mesotherapy has developed a lot in the realm of sports and especially among young patients. Their reactions are much more dramatic and efficient as compared to the elderly. Mesotherapists consider they are still conventional medical doctors. It is reassuring to patients. To leave conventional medicine is to leave the reimbursements of the National Health Service, to leave academic medicine and to take the risk of being misjudged. What a pity! They miss out considerably. This way they are not making any progress in advancing the promising future of their technique.

For a long time, I was convinced I practiced the same as mesotherapists because I put small doses of drugs in my injections.

In 1985 I became a member of the French Mesotherapy Society. I was happy to belong to this society, an established and recognised one.

My practice evolved over time into neuromedicine. But I couldn't talk about it, technically speaking. As long as I hadn't written the conceptual bases for this new medicine, I could only be considered a mesotherapist.

I was convinced that my research would be a useful contribution, even an indispensable one. So for a long time I tried to persuade my colleagues in mesotherapy of their rational foundation. I even tried to align myself with possible allies. I visited many known contemporary mesotherapists. This is how I met Dr. Perrin, a well know Parisian mesotheapist. He seemed to understand me, but was unable to agree with me.

Dr. Ballesteros, with an initial training in homeopathy, was keen on the body energy concept and the Kirlian effect. The latter consisted of recording on the feet a radiation which could be captured on a photographic plate.

This recording was pretty characteristic of the individual's energy levels and one could visualise the traces of fatigue.

I could have written Daniel Ballesteros, who strayed away from the French Mesotherapy Society, but I surmised that he was not my mentor but a "master". It was consequently impossible for him to accept my theories because he was obsessed with his own, which I thought to be incomplete. This school studied body energy without any connection to nervous system functions. As for what interested me, it was the nervous system as a daily actor in everything that happens in the body.

Didier Mréjen, another influential doctor, developed a technique that he called "Punctual Systematised Mesotherapy". It was, in my view, mesotherapy adapted for acupuncturists. With his work, he succeeded in creating his own school. The doctors who practised his technique felt that his theory gave them support, where they were empirical and subjective. Dr. Mréjen gave them a procedure backed by a conceptual construct. As for me, I did not propose a technical procedure but a theoretical basis. However, it wasn't needed because they all agreed that mesotherapy was microdose conventional medicine. Period.

I was also interested in the works of Dr. Walker of Clermon-Ferrand. He presented his results of treatment of recurring infections using micro-injections with a polyvalent vaccine much employed at the time called "Ribomunyl".

I was obstinate. I went to Dijon, Clermont-Ferrand, Besançon, Cannes, to all the mesotherapy congresses where I found my "friends". But I was beside their school, not one of them. I tried to show them how through the rolling palpation technique, one could locate pain or no pain. In doing this, I became too aggressive for them, a foreigner. Even today I feel they don't understand me. They see me as a mutant, maybe not dangerous, but like one of those "enlightened" doctors that one finds in medicine. I explore areas of interest that are absolutely out of their medical sphere of operations.

I reached the climax of this conflict at the Strasbourg Conference in 2008. A very impressive one with about 400 mesotherapist in attendance. This goes to show how flourishing mesotherapy is and how well it is doing.

I took the podium and, as usually evoked my theme: Microdosae Conventional Medicine or Re-educative neuromedicine? It was a big flop as usual. Undauntedly I pounded my fist on the podium and 400 faces looked at me with indifference, even reprobation. At the end of this conference, I approached the professor in charge of scientific matters. I asked him why he didn't give me his support and a chance for validation of a truth that was an interesting one. He responded that he knew well the limits of mesotherapy. For, to him, post-operative pain from a thoracotomy done to carry out four or five Coronary Artery Bypass Grafts could not be relieved without drugs.

Mesotherapy in this case, was of no point. I tried to explain to him that a severe pain that persists in post-operation confirms by its intensity and duration the existence of an enormous neurologic deficit already in place. One must start mesotherapy before the operation to treat early on this pain state, which is pre-existent and easy to show through the rolling palpation technique. A preventive session could reactivate a neurologic capacity locally, which would limit the postoperative pain.

I told him about one of my patients. A 35-year-old woman was exhausted from a Guillain-Barré syndrome which resulted in motor deficits. She consulted me. She didn't have any feeling of bladder plenitude so needed regular urinary catheterizations. By my neuromedical treatment, in 6 months, she recovered much of her bladder autonomy. In 40 days, she had already lost the tiredness and had re-started walking.

In the case of this young woman, traditional medicine and mesotherapy would have only treated the bladder. In contrast, I worked on the holistic picture, without which in the long run she would not have regained her autonomy. I was unaware that on choosing a case of neurologic bladder, I was trodding on his own territory as a Professor of Rehabilitation, so he simply refused to discuss it.

Nevertheless, mesotherapy is still a valid medicine, especially concerning the treatment of pain, sports injuries and among young patients. It finds its limits in tired out older patients.

What does one do when it doesn't work? You have to reconstruct the tired out patient. Me, I know how to do this!

I learned that I needed to leave mesotherapy. If it was coherent in itself and in line with conventional medicine, it was incoherent with respect to what I judged to be an enlightened approach to medicine.

But I wasn't either in the conventional medicine school of thought. But this didn't mean I would adhere to other theories such as that of the energy people who argue for a psychogenic view, which I felt was a cul-de-sac. Energy belongs to the total body. One cannot box it up in spirit or psyche. Those that speak of "psychoenergy" confuse energy with willpower. This willpower confronts the limitations of adaptability. You can change the capacity to rebound (the energetic potential) and give it more tonus through self-work, but it is a given that your limits stem from your neurologic rebound potential.

I think I am one who has most used "mesotherapy" for over thirty years. I have treated from 30 to 35 patients per day, so about 200,000 sessions. Nonetheless, I decided to quit looking obstinately for recognition among my meso-therapist colleagues and to break off from their obtuse school.

I was persevering with my research...

3 A brief history of medical thought

"I ask the question: 'If ever there only existed one disease?'"

Five centuries before our era, Hippocrates gave "dignity" to man. He developed a medical thought that departed from magic or religion, which until then was the basis for medical care. In those olden days, diseases that were badly defined appeared as an expression of a demonic presence that needed to be exorcised. Hippocrates viewed illness as a natural phenomenon. The weakness in the pharmacopeia of the time incited him to support at best a dependence on natural forces in each body to be cured. This man of art tried to do this through his advice on health that only a conscientious foreman could follow. Also, Hippocrates only cared for citizens, not slaves. It was not a problem of money but of liberty. Who cared for those men that were not free?

In the Second Century AD Galen, philosopher and doctor, took up the theories of Hippocrates and systematised them. His works were very influential until the Renaissance. According to him, the body was controlled by four "humours": the blood, the bile, the mucus, and the black bile. And the "pneuma" or "spiritus" in Latin, "souffle" in French, and "breath" in English. According to Galen this breath of life was an extract of the lungs from inhaled air, before being sent to the heart to undergo combustion. Called "vital spirit" in this way, it was infused into the blood, contributing to the circulation. When it reached the liver, "vital spirit" was transformed into "natural spirit";

and this latter governed nutrition. When it reached the brain, it was changed into animal spirit "psychic pneuma", which transported information derived from the five senses. Disease was then caused by disorders of the "humours" or of the breath.

With the Renaissance, humanists questioned these truths. But the Universities opposed new research for a long time, thinking that all was explained by Galen. We saw the increase of experimental studies, mostly in the domain of Anatomy, which up until then was limited by the religious ban on dissections. This initial progress was all the same framed by religious morays, which considered man a sacred creature and the life of man as a gift from Heaven.

Thus each advance in medicine had to allow a closer view of God. Didn't Ambroise Paré, half-cleverly half-modestly said of one of his patients: "I treated him, God cured him"?

At this time, they were looking for a principle that could link up all the organs. After the vital breath, they gave priority to the heart. The life of man existed thanks to the heart and the vascular system, which replaced breath: to feel unwell at heart, heart racing, heartburn, etc.

The scientific progress in the 18th Century swept away this scholarly empiricism. Little by little, the spirit of science influenced medicine. Diseases became better codified. Their origin ceased to be attributed to a spontaneous event. Through his experimental methods, Claude Bernard defined man as an organ system. He was much interested in digestion, where he discovered the criteria of normal physiology. One could then distinguish the disease from the normal state.

In the 20th Century, technology reinforced this tendency towards mechanical and chemical medicine. This effectiveness exists at the price of a very specialized compartmentalization of the body, which still leaves up God to synthesize it all.

For the 21st Century, I formulate a new hypothesis: the nervous system is the essential reality in all diseases and will concern medicine of the future.

This is not to replace "modern" medicine or to oppose it, but to complement it through new approaches. In the long run, these approaches will not subtract from its value but take from it a usurped predominance.

Western medical thought concentrates on quantifiable matter. Eastern medical thought is holistic. It does not separate the body and spirit. In fact, there exists something that is in neither one nor the other, but links them together. This is energy which one must now view as a functional neurologic system. It acts autonomously in its management of events of life. It constitutes a reservoir of rebound potentials in service of the spirit and the organs it either stimulates or inhibits. So one must now accept a triple vision of man, not a binary one: body, spirit and functional neurological system (neuroenergy).

I can assure you that over thirty years of medical practice has demonstrated that this part of our nervous system, not considering the cognitive reality of spirit, has a major impact on our diseases. This interactive behavior is expressed not in a linear way but an exponential one, and it is sometimes responsible for irrecoverable threshold ruptures.

I conclude that one's functional equilibrium is the guarantee for good health. Its capacity for adaptation may be maintained by exercises of many types, either physical or psychological.

This hypothesis is the basis of neuromedicine.

The ideas of neuromedicine will diffuse into medical thought ineluctably. It rejoins the evolution of its Century, which favors individual liberty, the right of each person to good health and to assume the responsibility for it. It is a personal medicine.

Neuromedicine is a medicine of "all time". Thus it returns to a holistic approach that evokes the breath of life of Galen, which is revived in this audacious modern conception of medical thought.

Ancient medicine, without specific drugs, was also a holistic medicine. It had the tendency to favor methods susceptible to permit self-cure. Much unlike the bleedings and other local techniques very obsolete, neuromedicine is a powerful rehabilitation through microstimulations. It promulgates a better self-management of energy resources in the body, which allows for adaptation in each person.

The future of this new medical line of thought rests on the progress of the neurosciences. This is not really reassuring because the research is so far from the reality of the daily work of a General Practitioner.

Our clinical experience should guide the basic research because, after all, in fact, neurofunctional medicine preceded it. It necessitates consolidating their theories using real patients. When this link to the neurosciences is made, we will have an answer to the "how and why". In this, neuromedicine will certainly be a controversy with the adherents of a genetic theory of life. A real false debate in reality because man is composed of genetic make-up, cultural background, and his environment.

4 The neuroscientific hypothesis

"All scientific progress arises out of innovative and daring imagination."

Science does not answer the questions I have as a doctor, clinician and caregiver in neuromedicine. I know how to treat. But for the interpretation of my results and especially in order to communicate them, I have constructed theoretical models which allow to predict and to reproduce their achievements. This permits improvement of the treatment.

I have, therefore, developed a system that is comprised of the following notions:

1) Body functions

2) Holistic and local dimensions

3) Energy: fabrication, management of stock (the rebound capacity), regulation (arc reflexes)

4) The autonomic nervous system

5) Recording in memory

6) Rehabilitation and prevention

7) Hypothalamus

Body functions

One calls "functions" the various expressions elaborated by the body to ensure life and external relations.

These functions are linked to the different organs where they occur.

Internal functions include essentially digestion, respiration and the cardiovascular system, the kidneys and elimination of urine.

External functions allow the individual to interact with his environment: the five senses, speech, cognitive functions, motor functions, etc.

Cerebral functions are varied. They have a role in the co-ordination of the internal functions, but they also intervene in the interactions of external functions. The nervous system maintains coherence between all the functions.

Holistic and local dimensions

Our health is grounded by two principal phenomena that allow for a complementary harmony in the body.

1) Adaptation at a local level, responding to needs.

2) Survival instinct at the global holistic level.

In disease, there is a rupture of this harmony due to major stress. The exacerbated local problem becomes preponderant while the whole person tires out in search of equilibrium.

In this dramatic scenario, neuromedicine recreates the equilibrium by adding a violent acceleration through supplementary stress. One provokes a survival reaction which reinstates our whole well-being. One reconstructs a global unity where there was a conflictual dissociation between local and global levels.

Energy

- Fabrication

All the cells of the body make energy. All give life and represent, both isolated and together, an enormous stock of energy. Nerve cells called neurons have a very specific role to play. They concern "energy of life": They have the responsibility of managing the body in its entirety and also each function separately.

Our nerves transport energy thanks to an electric influx, which provokes at their extremity liberation of a substance called neuromediators that allow each function to occur.

Neurons are always in action. They adapt according to the organ's needs, even in excess but on the condition that they stay below a certain threshold. Above this threshold, the overactivity stops the energy flow and the body reaches its physiological functional limits. One's production of daily energy is very individual and quantitatively specific.

- Management of stock

The body requires each day a certain quantity of energy to perform basic functions such as respiration, thinking, emotivity, eating, working, etc...

Our lifestyle creates a daily energy consumption level that is regular and durable. This determines the amount needed for a day according to the production potential. There is, however, a maximum threshold.

If, on some days, we use much more energy, we put our body in jeopardy. The body adapts and creates a small debt of energy. If the energy spent is excessive and continues, the body tries to adapt, both at the organ level and the entire energy stock level.

If one eats too much, then the body will adapt without difficulty. But if one overeats for many days in a row, the digestive system will suffer and one's local and general condition will show signs of acute fatigue. If one overeats for months or years, durable energy debt is created, which can result in chronic diseases like arterial hypertension or diabetes.

Long-term excesses don't result in a linear expression but an exponential one. The body, trying to resolve the problem brings more and more overactive nerve centers into action. Then return to an equilibrium becomes problematic and uncertain.

One must admit that a large part of the daily energy stock is used in anatomic body functions. Nevertheless, besides this energy stock, there is no other. The ability to meet the excess needs can only come out of this stock. So it is important for one to be conscientious of his stock available in order to manage it best.

- Dynamics of the spring

The nervous system is a spring. If a physical or psychological demand is made on one, then the body reacts and adapts to this. The nervous system acts like a spring. If the demand is not too much, the spring will return to its initial position afterward without breaking. So the spring was sufficient. But if the demand is more significant, recuperation can take several days, so any further effort during this time is unwise.

Above a certain threshold, which involves both duration and intensity of the demands, the body becomes overcharged in an overloaded frozen state: disease occurs. This condition which one would think to be deficient, is really an adaptation, a respite for the body which feels in danger. Once disease starts, the spring recoils sharply in response to all the consequences of the disease on the body. To avoid a possible catastrophe, this spring remains operable and maintains an equilibrium where there still exists a potential that fights the disease. One is always surprised at the resistance of our spring. A patient smokes, overindulges, overworks, and yet he makes out ok.

If you efficiently remove the impact of disease with a drug, you decrease the tension in the neurologic spring. If you remove the presence of infection, you give back the neurologic energy. At this stage – and only at this stage, conventional medicine is a medicine of rehabilitation because it acts upon the spring by releasing it. But drug-related recovery is horizontal and temporary. Its protection does not affect the global future of the body. In chronic diseases or in certain recurrent conditions, there is a great possibility that the body succumbs to the disease once again as soon as the drug is stopped and the spring receives another demand on it.

In the course of our life, this spring ages: very effective and sensitive as a child, but less so as an older person. When the demands accumulate, it does not recharge itself. The spring has no more force. The organs of the body, each according to their specificities, make local adaptations. Organ functions are arranged in arc reflexes, which testify to the intense threat of fatigue that they can contribute to sustain.

- Regulation: the arc reflex

Management of all functions occurs according to needs via a neurologic loop. An organ is solicited by a nervous center. The impulse travels from center to organ, then from organ to center, bringing adaptive response. This is an arc reflex.

For cutaneous nerve receptors, the arc reflex adds to the response of sensitive nerves and amplifies the motor response induced by the nervous centers in the spinal cord: Burning of the hand causes one to remove it quickly. This is a reflex action.

Global fatigue decreases the central regulation, which is often an inhibiting one. It results in excessive and too long reflex responses. This is also true for emotions.

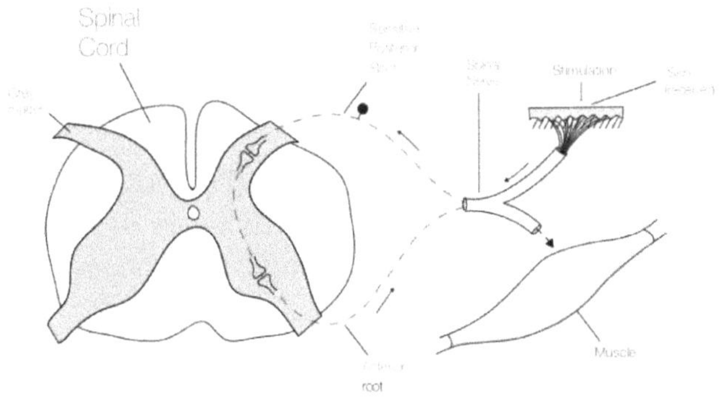

Neuromedicine re-equilibrates the functioning of arc reflexes through its treatment methods. This is particularly true at the cutaneous level. As we shall see, all disease states exacerbate the functioning of nervous circuits and have a repercussion on the cutaneous neurologic circuits in provoking hyper-reactivity.

Inversely, stimulation of a zone on the skin corresponding to a disease calms down the behavior of these loops. If, in an initial period of time, cutaneous injections aggravate the system (dramatization) by adding a "stress" to a "stress", they automatically decrease reflex hyperactivity in the spinal cord nervous centers (inhibition). The examination of the skin, which was so painful, becomes normal (analgesia).

The spring is released for a time. The reflex loop returns to its basal state.

Stocking in memory of conflicts

One calls "conflicts" all stress occurring in the body, whether physical or psychological in nature. In the course of our life, we generate all kinds of inner conflicts through our commitments, whether these are conscious ones or unconscious ones. Some of these conflicts are very significant and we continue to live with them unconsciously. They parasite our daily life being inscribed in active nervous circuits. We can't escape these conflicts. In the long run, we enter into a state of hyperreactivity, which renders any new conflict unbearable. Memory integration is the successful transition of a conflict into a habit, making future life experiences easier to live with. If this is done correctly, our daily life has no pending conflicts to deal with. Each new stress will find an adequate response, energy-saving in nature, thanks to information held in the cortex.

When significant stress is persistent or multiple, it can't be "digested", and it is not stocked in memory, so our feeling of well-being is impeded by the hormones responding to the stress. The accumulation of stresses not stocked away in memory leads to deep fatigue.

If you run without having any training, you rapidly enter into a stress situation in the body. You have pain, are out of breath, and generally out of energy and exhausted. If you insist, you provoke a rupture: a muscle disorder or tendon rupture or even heart failure. However, regular and progressive training sessions allow the body to put these situations into memory as they occur, and one becomes accustomed to the stress.

This example can be applied in the same manner to emotional stresses.

As it removes the local pain and/or emotional stress, treatment by neuromedical measures decreases the global requirement for adaptation, it gives back energy and allows for memory storage.

The autonomic nervous system

The autonomic nervous system responds to body needs. It especially acts on the heart and the vessels, the lungs and digestion. It regulates sensibility, muscle tonus and intervenes in mood states.

It is comprised of two nervous systems whose roles are often opposite ones: parasympathetic and sympathetic nervous systems.

For example, in the stomach, the parasympathetic vagus nerve (X cranial nerve) is responsible for the secretion of HCl after meals. It stimulates the muscles. In contrast, the sympathetic system relaxes muscles and provides muscle tonus for the upper sphincters (cardia) and lower ones (pyloric muscle).

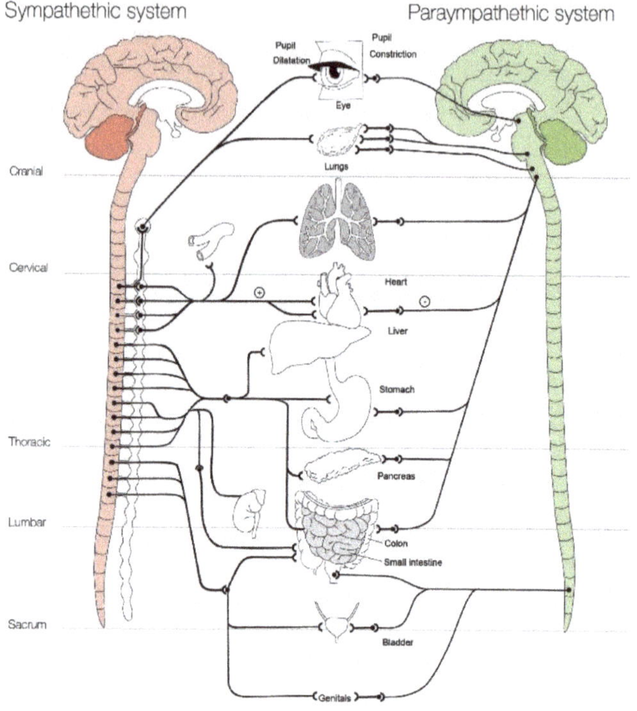

In the heart, the parasympathetic decreases the heart rate, while the sympathetic accelerates it. The latter also regulates blood pressure by its actions on smooth muscles of the blood vessels. The parasympathetic contracts bladder muscles and releases the smooth muscle sphincter, which allows for urination to take place. The sympathetic relaxes the bladder muscles (detrusor) and contracts the smooth muscle sphincter to ensure continence.

The sympathetic system is constantly delivering a direct effect. The parasympathetic system acts on occasion and in precise situations.

When one is in function, this favors the activation of the other one. Thus, in running a race, the increase in heart rate stimulates a return to a lower average heart rate when at rest

Rehabilitation and prevention

There are two ways to treat a sick body: either you replace or repair the sick part (conventional medicine, surgery), or you stimulate the body (rehabilitation).

In the first case, you treat the defective body as in an infection, and emotional or physical trauma, aging, etc. You do this using drugs for sickness or by resolving the problem through surgery.

In the latter case, you stimulate the body in order that the body reconstructs itself through the formulation of an internal response towards a self-cure. Either one gives support where there is deficiency (conventional drugs of substitution) or through re-education which renders the body competent again. Rehabilitative medicine intervenes on a local level but the readaptation that occurs is on a global central level. It allows a local recovery.

Of course, neuromedicine is a rehabilitative method that stimulates a readaptation by its entire action on the nervous system, both peripheral and central. Neurologic functional medicine addresses itself to minor and often recurrent diseases for which drugs have not been effective. This fact stems from the existence of "self-generating" loop reflexes. Untreated, this leads to gross fatigue and can be the start of an organic disease.

Multiple neurologic stimulations have a double action: a local action in suppressing minor diseases which most often evolve infraclinically (no symptoms); and a central action by regulation of stress phenomena that increase the capacity for adaptation of the organism.

This approach is preventive against the risk of reoccurrence and exacerbation of diseases.

Hypothalamus

At the center of neuromedicine is a central regulator of somatic functions of every kind: the hypothalamus.

It is at the crossroads of body sensibility and both neurologic and endocrine functions. It ensures homeostasis and, in effect, is the guardian of a permanent internal equilibrium without which life is impossible.

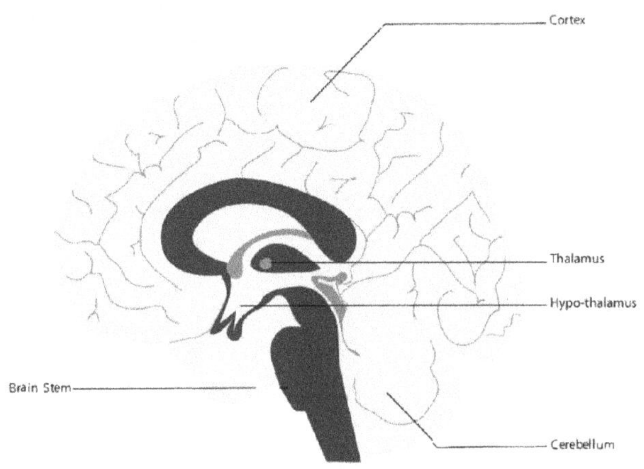

Disease occurs when homeostasis is threatened by an overcharged demand to adapt: the energy required is more than the available production of energy; the spring has reached its limits. The neurologic system is disturbed. The reflex loops exacerbate and fatigue the central responses. And the storage in memory of stresses is over-run.

This approach to disease challenges today's medicine's concept that is only focused on the organ and its lesions.

5 Organic or neurofunctional disease

"Body and nerves, a game of hide-and-seek."

Disease and patient

The ramifications of this neurological hypothesis cover a lot of conceptual differences between neuromedicine and contemporary medicine. Between disease and patient, local lesional states and local inflammatory states of a functional origin.

Nevertheless, these two worlds are finally complimentary and, in my opinion, are one and the same.

Medicine since the early days has concentrated on one of two poles. These have been emphasized differently according to country and over time. They are Disease and Patient.

In our time, modern medicine brings specific answers to cure diseases. They are effective. One cannot reproach this. All the better if we live in a world where our diseases have been controlled in great part and where life expectancy is long.

Its success derives from a complete knowledge of etiology.

We study the causes and consequences independently of the patient who is sick. The action of drugs authorises in fact, thinking that the patient is secondary. This is in part true for infections or acute diseases. But it is an error in chronic diseases or disorders of the aging where the absence of prevention leads to severe complications. For the doctor, disease is an abnormal condition which he needs to react to.

In my view, it seems today to be an intermediary step in which a patient finds himself for cultural, emotional reasons or just by being afraid of a change. It is also a question mark: What shall I do? Reject it or understand it? Understand why one is ill.

Disease in a patient results from an energy rupture, a poor adaptation that becomes worse. Patients have lost their inner equilibrium. This condition exists in a global energy dimension for which ancient remedies often address themselves to.

A cure is a return to equilibrium by the recovery of vital forces. Health is this newfound equilibrium that needs to be managed. So treatment and prevention go together at the same time.

Neuromedicine says the patient should commit to their quest for good health. It necessitates a thoughtful behavior and a certain philosophy concerning human relationships. In the face of grave events, regardless of religious beliefs, it must also bring a kind of spirituality into play, allowing liberation of the soul.

Notions of patient and disease cannot be separated. Against diseases, should we especially focus on the specific causes or rather a non-specific action where the body is asked to recover its equilibrium?

Doctors are interested in organic diseases. Here their modes of treatment are effective. This lesional conceptualsation is reinforced by laboratory examinations and imagery, which evidence presence of an organic lesion.

A fracture, an ulcer, a myocardial infarction are all organic lesions. The tissues or organs show visible alterations or lab results show anomalies. Conversely, functional anomalies don't always have lesions but just minimal inflammation.

However, many doctors think the contrary. For them, there cannot exist a functional anomaly without a lesion.

Neurogenic pain could convince them of their error, but they deny it. They say that the lesion is so small it can't be visualised, so-called neurologic microlesions. But can one explain how in certain cases, zona pains persist for many years when since long ago, the cutaneous lesions have disappeared?

We attribute certain leg pains to edema and migraines to intracerebral dilatations of vessels. But isn't it the converse that occurs? Isn't it rather the edema and venous anomaly that are secondary to an irritational condition and a neurologic functional failure?

Let's take the example of sciatica. This organic disorder is due to the irritation of a spinal nerve root, often after alteration of an intervertebral disk. Later, the presence of a discal hernia can complicate matters by compressing the nerve root between the two vertebrae. This situation provokes pain and muscle cramps at the lumbar level that projects to the lower limb.

Sciatica begins with spontaneously recoverable pain (or with the aid of drugs) for a short duration. When this becomes exacerbated and continues over several months, we enter into a chronic condition.

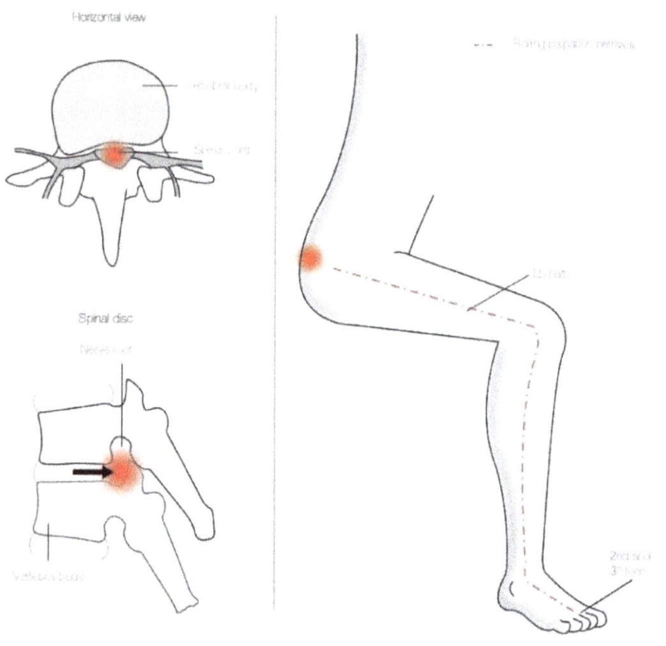

In an organic approach, mild pains that regress quickly are neglected. If symptoms persist or in case of acute exacerbation, a surgical operation will be carried out. The surgeon cuts out all or part of the disk to eliminate the compression on the nerve root, and thus remove the disk-root conflict.

Surgeons aren't obliged to see a relationship between local lesion and chronic inflammatory disease which caused the disk to bulge (thus the hernial complication). I call this inflammatory state a neurofunctional anomaly. The inflamed tissues over a long time are stressed by daily activities which self-maintain the inflammation. In the long run this favors vertebral disk degeneration and risks of severe decompensation.

I consider that these processes are of progressive occurrence in the disease and that they are caused by neurologic anomalies of the regulation of inflammation, of pain and of muscular tonus.

Pain is much intensified by physical efforts, but in time the physical causes have a lesser impact as compared to the fatigue and stress which play a preponderant role.

This repeated pain plays the role of a semaphore signaling sporadically flashes of alarm. In the ten years which precede a major crisis, the patient has not understood the "reason" for these signals.

This is how, at a slow pace, our diseases get underway. The reasons often come down to this period that precedes the crisis.

Neuromedicine integrates the local phenomenon into the history of the patient.

Jonathan, 20 years old, is in masonry training. The job he has to do is too hard for his unprepared body. He has pain in his back and lots of anxiety because he doesn't think he can finish training. He calls on, even more, his capacity to adapt because he is stressed-out psychologically. Moreover, if Jonathan has emotional problems, smokes or goes to bed late, we have all the ingredients for a very bad scene. In a first instance, the hypothalamus programs an appropriate response to compensate for local deficits: "Are you lifting too heavy sacks? Don't worry, I will send you little soldiers and program you for a few days so you can still carry them without a problem."

But he exceeds this quota, and little by little, he enters into a spiral of failure. He decompensates first locally by strong reflex cramps that accompany his pain. A lumbar disc is affected. This could remain as is; in a sensitiveness to physical strain. But any additional excess effort could lead to an acute discal hernia. This, in turn, will irritate, then compress the nerve root and consolidate. This is the vicious circle of disease.

All diseases are explained by this example of a young man who created a discal hernia in himself.

The organic stage is the last one in a "neurofunctionallde-ficient" condition, which has evolved for a long time. Neuromedicne does not compete with conventional medicine in acute diseases. For the most part, it intervenes before this by prevention. It treats both local and central neuro-functional deficits. It also addresses itself to the psychological aspects of the patient. Thus, these three comprise a global treatment of the patient. Neuromedicine is a holistic medical science and art of healing.

6 Principles of neuromedicine

"I scan with my fingers I inject to stimulate I reset the spring I create a future."

Neuromedicine is based on specific exploratory techniques of the body and perfectly codified treatment.

Techniques of body exploration: the rolling palpation technique

- A diagnostic tool

Neuromedicine is based on the rolling palpation technique which interrogates the "unconscious body", diseases before they actually appear. The rolling palpation makes pain readable by our fingers before the appearance of symptoms or any lesions. It "scans" the body in order to discover not organic profiles but neurofunctional ones. Without even speaking to the patient, I can evidence zones of suffering and indemn zones that the skin demonstrates in the absence

of any conscient knowledge of the patient. This discloses to patients the existence of an "unconscious" of the body just like the unconscious that Freud disclosed of the mind.

These zones where the body shows a rupture of its equilibrium allows us from the very start to evidence neurofunctional disorders and to obtain a picture of their clinical reality. In this way, one perceives places where the patient is in conflict with himself and also elsewhere, where there are no conflicts. All pathologies are found through the rolling palpation technique. It is a tool of both diagnostic and predictive analysis.

So there are three realities sometimes discordant to reckon with: the complaint of the patient, the results of various exams, and the infallible pain revealed by the rolling palpation technique. Sometimes there is a contradiction between what the patient says and what is found on examination. When patients describe their pain with respect to their condition, they always feel maximum pain.

The rolling palpation technique allows me to get more information on pain. By my touch, I can get an idea of the nature of their suffering, its severity and age, in light of the feeling of the patient when this is excessive with respect to clinical data.

Perception can be modified as a function of the present circumstances of the patient. A relaxed person will have a less exaggerated sensibility. Moreover, in a man who just ran a marathon one detects very little pain on palpation because his body is inundated with endorphins. Conversely, someone who has not slept has exaggerated reactions. Neuroleptic treatment also perturbs the rolling palpation results.

Thus, the indications obtained by rolling palpation must take in to account pre-existing conditions.

- The rolling palpation technique

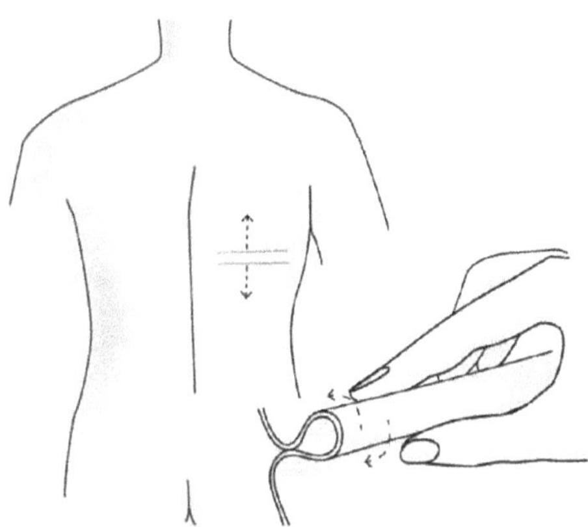

Rolling palpation is a dynamic exam of the skin. By squeezing the skin between the thumb and the index finger, one crates a roll of skin pressing on the dermis. One rolls along the skin from low to high, from high to low, and/or laterally. Thus, one evaluates the cutaneous structures and the way the skin is attached to deeper tissues. One finds supple zones, normal.

Or more rigid and thick zones where pain is sharper. One notes the contractures of the muscles of the skin, which makes harder the rolling between the fingers, and zones that are "crunchy" indicating older zones of suffering.

I have only based my theories from my daily intake of patients. You have knee pain, I use the rolling palpation tool.

You have liver dysfunction, I use the rolling palpation tool. You have neck pain, I use the rolling palpation technique. If you don't have back pain, I find nothing abnormal using the rolling palpation technique. If you have a sprained ankle and pain, I look for congestion over the cutaneous dermatome of L5. And there you have pain on palpation. In fact, sprained ankle affects the external lateral ligament and creates a reflex pain in the nerve from the buttock to the ankle. Treatment will be applied all along this nerve.

The rolling palpation technique reveals the neurological reality by integrating a pathology with the central nervous system.

The injections

Neuromedicine involves stimulation of the reflex arc as defined by zones revealed by the rolling palpation technique. In my experience, this stimulation is more powerful than massage or acupuncture.

One uses multiple intradermic injections. These act as microstimulations whose intensity varies as a function of the surface treated, the depth, and the number of injections, as well as the nature and quantity of the drugs injected. These intradermic stimulations can be either superficial or deeper. One can establish a quantified treatment protocol, then carry it out.

My base product is magnesium diluted in saline solution. This cannot be considered as a drug. The presence of Magnesium magnifies the local stimulation and makes it last longer. This is not mesotherapy because I do not inject a specific drug and also because I am working with the body as a whole.

Dermatomes, meridians, and the nerve plexus

I have been working on establishing a map of the dermatomes for over 30 years. These are precise systematised thin nerve maps that thicken and spread out in the presence of pathology causing neurologic disturbances in a particular point along the dermatome. Whenever a pathology arises and there seems to be a thread of pain, there is actually a large ribbon of pain as described by a zone in the dermatome.

Starting at the vertebrae, the dermatomes design circles that are superimposed on each other at the trunk level and are distributed in a regular and linear fashion out to the extremities of the limbs. These are identical in aspect going to deep tissues to membranes that englobe the bones or the viscera (skin, subcutaneous fat, muscles, and periosteum). The rolling palpation technique easily evidences these dermatomes by detection of lines of cutaneous hypersensibility even in the absence of any pathology.

We call segmentary the relationship between the dermatomes and the nerve centers of the spinal cord. The supra-segmental level concerns the central brain. I have noted that there isn't a painful zone in the knee without a projection to the spinal column (segmental level).

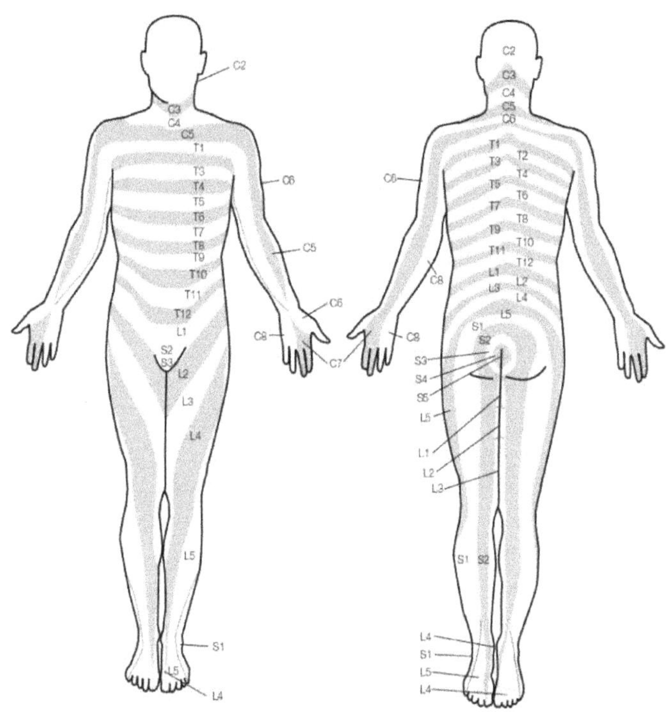

Then I realised that one could not suffer from lumbar pain without a cervical projection (supra-segmental level). These two levels are linked by the meridians, vertical lines like those in acupuncture. These are sensitive to the rolling palpation technique and mix with the dermatomes at the internal surface of the limbs.

All pathologies are also defined as a function of the nerve plexus which I have found to be P1 cervical plexus, P2 thoracic plexus, P3 visceral plexus, and P4 sacral plexus.

Let me give you an example. People eat way too much at Christmas. They are going to have a hepatic congestion, which will cause suffering on the right in P3 at the visceral level. This irritation radiates down to produce lumbar pain or up to produce shoulder pain.

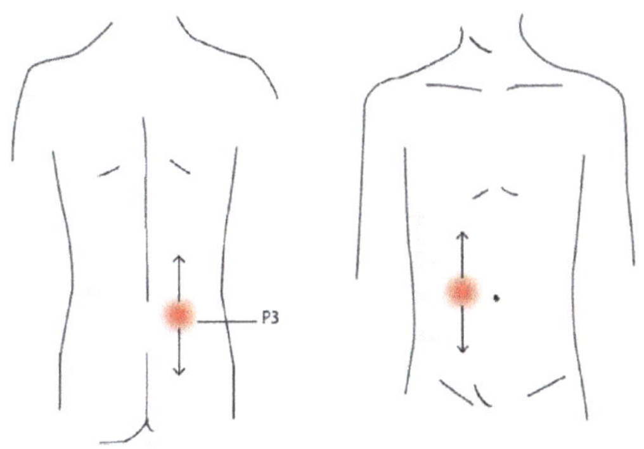

The 4 phases of each session: stimulation, sideration, re-action, adaptation – (SSRA)

In each session of neuromedicine there is a series of four phases: stimulation, sideration, reaction, adaptation.

Based on the repetition of this sequence, once a week depending on the need, healing occurs.

The first step is that of stimulation by injections (Day 1).

The second step is the time of sideration. Just after the injections, when the patient leaves the office, they are in a second stage, a subliminal state like that can be found in sophrology. They mistakenly go the wrong way when they leave the room. They feel "funny" like if they were in cotton and say they are in a little less pain.

The third step is that of the reaction (Day 2), which occurs habitually the second day. It can last some hours, sometimes rarely some days. Patients feel very lethargic and sometimes feel a painful exacerbation.

The Fourth step is that of healing (Day3), which I call a time of adaptation. Cure is of course suppression of symptoms, but if possible, also the capacity of the body to keep the symptoms away.

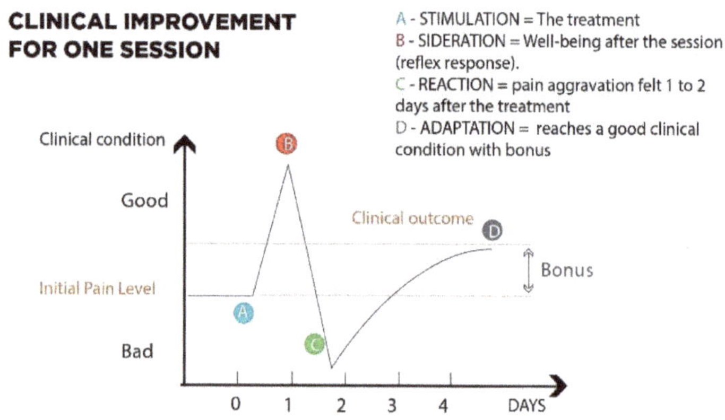

With equal stimulation, the reaction to it is not the same according to each body's threshold. Someone at ten years old does not have the same threshold as someone at 20 or 50 years old. And these thresholds must be constantly reviewed because in the course of treatment new equilibriums are obtained.

When a patient with a chronic disease is taken under treatment, i.e. States of pain more than three months old, one notes that the thresholds change. After the Second session there is no more sideration. Reaction time, which is usually major after this session, fades out until it disappears. Cure occurs slowly, sometimes in 40 days. In other words, through this treatment, I successfully created a deep modification in the behaviour of the organism.

A psychological dimension

My own experiences in psychotherapy contributed to my research. I am neither Lacanian, Jungian or Freudian. I merely understood that when one lets go of all his problems, he makes a step towards neurologic reconstruction. I learned that when a patient wept during a session, his progress was much faster. When one understands the causes of a rupture of equilibrium one can recuperate what was lost.

In understanding this phenomenon I infused into my treatment not only an empathetic approach to console and reassure patients but a complementary therapy of rehabilitation. I treated my patients not only in body but in spirit. If a patient is exhausted by either a somatic or affective conflict, the nervous system is always involved. Furthermore, emotional events play a major role on a neuroenergetic level.

In neuromedicine one associates body and mind because one acts on the global energy status.

Timing

Timing is an essential aspect of my work. In neuromedicine all restarts from zero because time is an attribute of pathology. Timing is especially a dimension of cure.

- Three days to cure a recent episode

A session of physical exercise too strenuous will require three days to get back to normal. Go see a bonesetter: it takes three days. Go see an osteopath or a mesotherapist: it takes three days. Three days also for a session of neuromedicine. By three days, I mean Day 1 it is the injections session, Day 2 the following day. And Day 3 you are reborn.

- Forty days to make the change

In the instance of an acute painful episode, a symptom of an old and deep pain, one can care for successfully and rapidly with a drug or a manipulation. However, this is not the end of it or the patient's history. How can one envisage an instant cure for an ancient event(s)?

In order to care for patients properly, one must put their pain into the perspective of their history. I must convince them to adhere to a treatment over an adequate duration.

Neuromedicine can, in other words, reorient the patient in his world. It relativizes the moment and gives back time to time... in 40 days. A Biblical reference that I find fascinating. The Bible was written by men in times when man understood time... Man in those days knew that a change occurred in 40 days. In other terms to rid the patient of nervous system parasites and allow for adaptation, it takes 40 days.

Many chronic pathologies of over 3 months duration require such a time to resolve themselves. It's the time of deep calming down, that of change.

- Six to eighteen months to rehabilitate

The nervous system reacts, calms down and reconstructs itself over time. Neurological disorders like algodystrophy – a disease of the sympathetic nervous system that is characterised by pain and stiffness that occurs after traumatic injury – evolve over six to eighteen months before stabilising.

Neuromedicine can gain time for these pathologies, but it does not permit an escape from the physiological reality. I obtain a clear improvement in the first month in chronic disorders. Nevertheless, I know that a complete cure often requires eighteen months.

- Give oneself time to accept inescapable life events

To give oneself time is to accept natural events.

Accept, for instance, that a mother is old, a sign of the nearing of a natural end of life. In spite of this, a son or daughter tends to spontaneously hope for the survival of their mother and deny the inescapable end. This makes them enter into a psychological state of pathological emotional denial and fear.

In neuromedicine I try to break away my patients from a negative view of aging. I try to help them give value to the time left to live. This is giving back to them a "future".

When I say, "Give yourself time," this means: "Discern events according to universal problems." This is difficult because it has to be learned. In reality, a good education should promote that: program an individual to give it time, regardless of the shocks and insults in life.

7 Five essential indications

"Rumpes arcum si semper tensum tenuis."

"The arc ruptures if it is always kept tense."

Neuromedicine has proven its efficiency for treating pain, regulation of muscular tone, vasomotor phenomenon, inflammation, immunity, and mood.

These functions, which constantly exist in a basal condition, can be modified in case of disturbances regardless of their origin. They are under the direct influence of the central nervous system and constitute a local non-specific response to a particular affected organ. Their functioning remains very sensitive to the general potential for adaptation.

Pain

- Making sense of pain

Pain is the most common complaint of patients. Although still read lots of articles on pain, although I follow efferent and afferent pathways, although I know nerve calibers, spinal and in-brain nerve center localization, in these articles I could never find the reality of pain that I encountered on a daily basis. The pains that I treat are unpredictable and obey their own laws. When I am confronted with them, I see myself as a snake charmer who doesn't make the mistake of thinking that they dominate that which always remains an adversary. In the snake, there is something nonreducible, for which one needs to reckon with. It's the same for pain. A law is inscribed in each patient and for each pain that we must learn to decipher.

What a disappointment when the radiological films demonstrate an insufficiently important cause with regard to a significant pain! So we construct a simplistic theory whereby the consequence (disease) hides causes that existed for several years.

Right away we look for an organic or mechanical etiology. Nevertheless, we vaguely feel that this pain shakes us up deeply, that it brings us back to something emotional and fundamental.

What unconscious and disquieting self-questioning lie behind all these symptoms?

Our pains often have a hidden aspect. They never occur at random and always when being fed up becomes a tsunami that overwhelms and submerges the neurological dikes. Then we are no longer protected.

They are global in nature and their causes are a mixture of current and past traumatic insults. Furthermore, these events which are not yet recognised in cortical memory prevent the body from adapting, which favors emotional reactions and delays healing.

Not having found a satisfactory explanation for my patients in all my readings, I tried to construct an algorithm coherent with all my clinical observations. This can be criticised, not acknowledged, but no other true explanation

can be suggested because in this domain research is incon-
clusive.

Nevertheless, there are several points which need to be considered:

1) the local clinical perspective, a very evident one, is only half the story of the pain process. Behind this one finds the true story, especially in chronic diseases;

2) the major role played by the nervous centers in the spinal column which inhibit pain sensations (Gate Control);

3) the presence of a basic status of pain (sensibility) inhibited constantly by an anti-pain tonus. This can be shown by rolling palpation pressure evidencing existence of pain "without the patient feeling his pain". This inhibition disappears if a physical or psychological shock occurs there.

Exceeding a certain threshold level of stimulation, the pain influx reaches the superior nervous centers, and a double response occurs: a specific response which analyses and compares with respect to the cause, and a non-specific response in centers responsible for the management of stress.

- Taking care of the pain

Often, supportable pains are neglected. One assigns to them an insignificant cause and hopes that they go away. However, to neglect these pains generates a risk of eventual establishment of a chronic disorder. So in alternation we have periods of fatigue, hyperactivity and exacerbated sensitivity.

My role is to explain: "Pathology is a return to the law. It is often evidence of a lack of respect for oneself." I am therefore called upon to remotivate the patient. I have to consider their recent or past history both physical and emotional. I must push them to surpass their usual limits by a positivist proposition: "Me, I believe you can." A shoulder problem? It is obvious that we are always going to find an inf lammed tendon to treat, an acromio-clavicular conflict to care for, etc. The patient will feel better. But that doesn't solve the global problem of the patient's fragility. Besides, the shoulder problem may be resolved, but either they will have it again in three months or they will hurt elsewhere. This is why neuromedicine doesn't stop with treatment of the shoulder alone. It takes into account all the suffering in the areas found on rolling palpation which are involved here. The vertical lines translate the presence of these pains in a global neurologic dimension while the horizontal lines concern vertebral pains that are difficult to dissociate from those of the shoulder.

At the start of treatment neuromedicine attenuates pain locally. It causes a kind of analgesia. Pain which is still felt.

It seems "dispersed", as patients often exclaim. And on rolling palpation after treatment the pain has disappeared. But the patient declares they still feel it. This dissociation of central-local is systematically present as if the central trace of the pain was dissociated with its organic basis and evolved at different speeds over time. The physical sensation only shows up later in the mind. The local relief of pain liberates the upper central nerve centers of an exhausting conflict and can in time re-create the status of no pain. At the end of 40 days, to their surprise, despite their initial doubts, the patient discovers they feel no pain, feeling healed instead.

It is difficult to convince a patient that pain often is not serious. Patients dramatize their pain because it is underscored by their history. They are exhausted, caught up in the theatrical performance of their own existence.

Even if the snake charmer doesn't dominate the situation, he masterfully controls the snake. Likewise, the neuro-medical doctor subdues the pain, renders it "respectable", and gives it meaning.

Regulation of muscle tone

Muscle tone is an important basic function.

Our muscles are never entirely at absolute rest even when we sleep. Muscles constantly maintain our various postures and prepare for any subsequent movement. They remain ready to contract in response to an order either conscious or reflex. The reaction is sometimes maximal when an individual's safety is threatened.

This state of continuous vigilance of the motor system necessitates a minimal automatic functioning of the responsible nerve centers. They are themselves subjected to a global regulation capacity of the body in order to maintain and regulate them.

Each individual is constantly undergoing muscle contractions which originate in our daily activities. Physical and emotional stress are resorbed by them. Below a certain threshold, these contractions are not felt and disappear spontaneously.

In important physical or other use, a muscle contraction of variable severity can appear and last until provoking, for example, a torticollis or a lumbago. In the case of exhaustion, this function is exacerbated and frequent severe contractions occur permanently. Joints become stiff. These muscular contractions are thusly a part of the clinical picture in chronic disorders such as arthritis or fibromyalgia.

When there is no pain, these nevertheless symptomatic states result from a failure of the system and are not adequately considered in conventional medicine. But they are aways accompanied by muscle contractions in the skin which are so easily evidenced by rolling palpation. Not only that but they disappear as soon as the first injections are made. One measures in this case the effectiveness of neurofunctional treatment.

In some severe diseases where muscle tone is considerably elevated, we speak of spastic hypertonia. I am referring to Parkinson's Disease and the sequalae of neurologic pathologies such as hemiplegia.

Neuromedicine does not presume to replace conventional medical treatment but be used in synergy with it by decreasing significantly muscle contractions and pain. In the long run, one can hope for a better quality of life for the patient and even to slow down the evolution of the disease.

Neuromedicine acts in the same way in cases of congenital cerebromotor diseases where the patient is confined to a wheelchair in positions of hypertonia and any movement is not allowed. Blockages of adult patients could be avoided early in childhood before any uneducable postures occur.

Muscle hypertonia, like pain, is evidence of a deeper problem. To eliminate hypertonia, both mild and severe ones, is to provide the patients with a comfort of life they couldn't even imagine before. Neuromedicine compensates for these tensional states through better regulation of basic muscle tone.

Arteriovenous muscle tone and inflammation

For the veins and capillaries, there exists a basic functioning. The blood pressures are such in our lower limbs that without this tone we would have permanent edema and varicosities. This tone is indispensable in "homo erectus".

According to individual condition and age, the exhaustion of this function occurs, and can be quite early in some. The appearance of varicose veins is the sign of it. Often quite localised in the beginning, these show that a deficient neurofunctional condition is present which lets the muscles of the veins become atonic; they dilate passively. Traditionally these conditions are treated with venous sclerosis or removal, notwithstanding that they are recoverable for a long time by the stimulation of the arteriovenous tone.

Varicose veins spread out according to the dermatomes and are found from high to low in the lower limb. They are found in precise zones such as the external or internal surface of the thigh or calf with for any particular vein with alternation of healthy and diseased portions. This initial piecemeal aspect shows that the causal agent is not just high blood pressure spanning along the whole vein, but certainly a localized neurofunctional disorder.

The lesions remain in this dispersed fashion for quite a long time until the final decompensation occurs. Then a generalized varicose state settles, accompanied by fibrosis, varicosis, edema and ulcers. Here more than before, since the surgical cure is no longer indicated, neuromedicine has its role to play. It blocks the negative feedback of pain provoked by the cutaneous lesions in the whole of the spinal cord centers. The medullary centers when discharged of this neurologic overload permit a global improvement of all the lesions present.

Arteriovenous tone is also involved in the capillary circulation or microcirculation whose poor functioning results in edema. It accompanies in a systematic way inflammatory states especially as soon as a lesion appears, such as in an ankle sprain.

An active neurologic regulation is in place which limits the spread and number of lesions. Edema occurs when either there is disappearance or inhibition of the basic venous tone. A traumatic injury, an infection, or any other pathology causes inflammatory enzymes to be liberated which creates a loop reflex that renders all treatment ineffective.

I have had the opportunity to treat localised edemas, called idiopathic ones, because it seemed there was no cause. Those that I treated followed a precise path of L5 and essentially were found over the toes and the front of the foot. The swelling was about 3 or 4cm high, palpable, and not painful. Re-education over these paths from the buttock to the foot passing via the external surface of the lower limb reduced the edema significantly. So here the neurologic origin is confirmed.

Immunity

Immunity proves each of us to be different. We are unique and fabricate defenses to conserve our autonomy. Loss of this autonomy is dangerous.

The immune response is elicited to ensure survival. It protects our internal systems from any external invasions.

All sorts of products, beneficial or toxic, enter our bodies. Some don't have any corporeal existence, like ideas... As for our common illnesses, the notions of bacteria and viruses are very familiar to us.

We live in symbiosis with this infinitely microscopic world. Digestion, for instance, cannot occur without the aid of commensal bacteria in our intestines which help in the absorption of food.

But there are limits to this coexistence. Our interior world is constantly on guard. All intruders are fought heartily and usually killed off. This combat is permanent. One can see it on a local level by the existence of tissular and cellular defenses of the skin and the blood and more broadly speaking by the actions of the nervous system.

So-called auto-immune disorders are often severe because the body is fighting it's own substance matter. Allergies also show up as an immunity problem as in excessive local reactions in asthma and rhinitis.

Neurostimulations cannot be expected to treat satisfactorily all these immune states, but they have showed a significant effectiveness in repetitive and less severe conditions such as rhinitis and otitis, bronchitis in the infant where asthma is often involved with the infection. Here the general condition of the patient plays a preponderant role. Its excessive and repeated responses end up with the exhaustion of the neurologic function in question. Then released are local reflex responses to any stimuli like cold or hot, wind, stress, and in an exacerbated fashion to viruses that are so frequently encountered in all the public places of association such as schools. It results in a firework of pain, congestion with or without draining and even fever.

It is an error to think of these infections as primary ones. They are just the consequence of a sometimes tragic acquired tissular incompetence, such as in the tonsils which are supposed to combat infection. In fact, they maintain a continuous local inflammatory state whose immune action has become nil in the absence of preventive treatment through neuromedicine or thermal baths. The removal of tonsils and/ or adenoids is beneficial at two levels: it deletes an organ which has become a supplier of disease and it takes pressure off an exhausted nervous system because it was incessantly involved. It even became deleterious in favoring itself inflammation and infection.

Immunity does not only concern ENT infections. It also concerns other locations such as the bladder and female gentalia where recurrent infections are common. Treatment of deficient neurologic states in the lombo-sacral region and the lower sites gives good results in association with a general treatment of relaxation.

The real disease is not the emergence of an acute state where antibiotic treatment remains useful, but the repetition over time of these states.

Stimulation by the injections renders efficient the neurologic loops again. Inflammations disappear and immune reactions occur again. It occurs without any exaggeration in an adaptive way.

Mood regulation

Mood like pain or arteriovenous tone calls for a basic central nervous system action. An aggressive mood was a means of survival in prehistoric times. It is the same in our modern societies even if they tend to soften and regulate the relations of man with his natural and social environment. We are aways in a defense posture against others. Bad mood is therefore a normal basic condition in order to come to grips with daily activities and cope with life in the industrialised 21st Century.

Trying always to perform perfectly at all cost without respite calls upon our capacities to adapt. It generates successively hyperactivity and exhaustion. At first, being productive constantly, we become stressed out. We don't realise the process of exhaustion that is evolving. The next step is the appearance of signs that hobble us: pain, insomnia, anxiety, and spasmophilia or even neurosis in more fragile patients. It might stay at this stage, but often a patient goes into burn-out or depression.

The neurologic phenomenon here too is self-generated because constantly repeated emotions prevent any return to an equilibrium. These maintain exhaustion at a deep level.

In this context, the so-called natural and physiological bad humor takes on a new dimension. The inhibition of the production of endorphins or other neurohormones provokes durable phenomena associated with difficulties of mood: irritability, aggressivity, anger, dejection, sadness, exhilaration or withdrawal.

These behaviours do not spontaneously drive these patients to consult a doctor. Patients think that it is in their personality or the normal consequence of existential difficulties. Many hide their mood disturbances in order to conform to society. Whatever the case may be, these repeated outbursts come from an internal disorder, and thus a deficit in global nervous adaptation.

In most cases, I treat for mood, the patient has come for a different problem. Antonio Damasio in his book "Theory of Body Markers" suggests that emotional history is recorded in the nervous circuits of the body. Without a body, emotions are impossible, he writes. One can surmise that these circuits are evidenced in rolling palpation.

So stimulations in neuromedicine treat the body manifestations of stress and create a stable and appeased situation. This permits over time an improved adaptation of mood.

Exhaustion: it links all the patients together

This is the link between all the patients who consult me.

When I speak of exhaustion, I am not thinking of the marathon runner at the end of his run, neither of a child who goes on holiday after a long school year, nor of a woman who just gave birth. These people will recover in a short time because their fatigue is specific and limited in nature.

The exhaustion which I speak of is durable. It is often ignored because the signs present are not necessarily important. It can manifest itself by a fatigue but most often by a hyperactivity which is not yet really felt as an agitation. In this period, rest is unbearable or refused.

This state often gets worse and decompensates following a difficult episode in life. The patient cannot spring back because his energetic account is rather empty. So this is now not a momentary excess of energy spending but a structural deficiency in the crediting of the account. The central neurogenetic pump defuses itself and merely applies a constant law under the circumstances, i.e. Minimal production of energy.

A functional neurologic threshold has been reached. This rupture cannot be detected by a lab test or a scan. This state is inscribed in the reality of the patients' life and from now on recorded in their history. It goes through periods of excitation and withdrawal which is more or less long. Their emotions explode at the slightest provocation. Their body is bombarded. The vertebral column and the digestive system are the scapegoats. The pain appears at the least increment of stress and endures.

Without a global energy management harmony is impossible. Behaviours become reflexive and uncontrollable, these excesses aggravate the exhaustion. Thusly, some buy some piece of mind in the form of addictions: tobacco, alcohol, over-eating for the mildest! Sexual activity also but it is often used up early.

All these behaviours are able to extract from their body some drops of pleasure but at a great price for these patients who are dissociated by a "global-local" rupture.

The most fragile are often the youngest who make an exit from the mainstream: depression, accident, disease. They enter into the pathological consequences of exhaustion.

In chronic diseases, medical drug treatment is only palliative. It muffles the consequences of stress and its local expression limiting in this way the negative feed-back of these states on the energy deficit. Indispensable rest only serves to gain time.

In fact, the neurologic debt is very significant and slow recovery will only be partial without "turbo". It's a question of threshold. Neuromedicine finds its true usefulness in these situations.

At the local and segmentary level of the spinal cord, a blockage of exacerbated neurologic reflex responses is involved. Thusly, superior nervous centers are relieved. A progressive desensibilisation allows the formation of global responses that are more and more appropriate. The treatment induces a slow increase of energetic potential which permits the organism to reconstruct following successive neurologic levels.

8 Die to live at Millau

"To be reborn tomorrow, one must die today."

The 100 Kilometers of Millau (62 miles)

- Each of us has an energetic potential

Like each participant, I go into this run armed with my muscles, my mental set and especially my neuroenergetic potential in response to stress. I set a goal of time for the run which necessitates a certain pace. What will be my capacity to hold up without a break in my pace which I have chosen?

- The risks taken

I know that an unadapted organism manifests itself by decompensations. These can be either minor or major, even mortal from a cramp to dehydration. If I don't want any cramps I must simply go slower.

If my heart is not adapted to this effort, instead of beating at a rhythm of 120/minute when I run, it will beat at 130-140/min. This is an additional factor in exhaustion.

The nervous system also governs the needs for water. If I sweat a lot, lose lots of water and salt, it will create deficits in me little by little. I run, and I need to furnish my muscles with more and more blood that they require. The problem is that there is less and less when I dehydrate.

This gradual inadaptation due to dehydration can cause a major cardiovascular insult.

- *My run*

The first part of the run goes pretty well up until the 27th kilometer, equivalent to a half-marathon. Then I felt suddenly tired, in difficulty and I maybe had a minor malaise. A small rupture. A sort of "little death".

I know what is going to happen: I begin to need glycogen. The insufficiency of my training is revealed in this manner.

At any rate, with these pains and this heaviness I am obliged to walk for 10 to 15 kilometers.

Then at Kilometer 40 I restart up! It goes better because I slowed down and recuperated energy. I finish my first loop in Millau before beginning the run to Saint-Affrique. On a hill, I am obliged to change my shoes which were too new. I think myself saved but in reality it was a big mistake: I stopped several minutes and leaned forward to put on my old shoes. This posture provoked an elongation of muscles already very overworked. I can't restart the run; I have cramps and horrible pains in my back and groin.

I had a second rupture, a new "little death" which could well have been the last stop. I persevered. I began to walk again slowly. Until I reached the flat...this passed.

On the flat, I tried to jog at 4-5 km/h. At the end of some meters sharp pains in my hips reappeared. Also, I decided to put an end to my run at the next revitalization station which I was approaching slowly. When I jog the pain reappears, but I have the feeling that I had been able to do 10 or 20 meters more before starting to walk.

200 meters later, I retried and my impression was confirmed. New try. 1 km later, and this time I run 100 meters more before these pains arrived and paralysed my advance. Each slowing down regenerated energy and lifted the stress.

I now start the descent. I felt a little bit better. At the revitalization station, the person who gave us the coffee advised me: "Whatever you do, don't lie down. Don't sit down. Don't rest. Have a coffee and continue to walk, that's all." I understand that a brutal stop would be a change in state susceptible to put a new stress on me that I might not be able to withstand.

I had to rest without stopping.

So I listened to him and continued.

I realised I was accelerating gradually: 6 km/h then 8km/h and finally 10 km/h. It was euphoria. In 30 minutes I found again my capacity to run. It was then that I caught up with Jean-Claude...

Jean-Claude is 64 years old and at that time I was 54 years old. He told me at the start that unlike the year before he wanted to run seriously and so without me. And now I was passing him. This nice man was advancing in the midst of a whirlwind of young women. I felt strong from my sudden rebirth. To this lovely man who was snobbish to me at first I exclaimed: "Listen, Jean-Claude, I will leave you with the women and write you from the finish line!".

I was beginning the Tiergue hill climb. 5 km at 5% incline. Deadly! At my level of training, one doesn't run up climbs. So I walked at 4-5 km/h. I was very cautious. After 2 or 3 km, all of a sudden I hear behind me a bloke that says: "Is it you, Jean-Francois? "It is my friend Jean-Claude who remarks: "We don't leave each other, eh? You'll see, we'll show them!"

We did the climb by walking: on the plateau, we gulped down a coffee without stopping. We descended the hill towards Saint-Affrique. We had another coffee. Again, we climbed uphill for 5km at 7 km/h. We are in good enough shape. I'm not dead anymore. I am, on the contrary, very vigorous and managing better my capacities.

The complicity, the sharing of the run with Jean-Claude decreased my stress. I inversed the polarity of my mood. From a suffering loser I became a winner.

One dies when one exceeds his capacity to fabricate energy. At a minute's time, I was either dying or not. In fact, I cannot do more than what my training will allow, but the neurologic capacities of survival always exists in us.

We are now about 4 or 5 km from the end. Jean-Claude says to me: "Jean-François let's speed up! "Because we economised our energy in the previous 40 km, we could do 8 -9 km/h. We started to pass lots of runners who were arriving at the end – at least they thought – Jean-Claude went into a sprint in the final 100 meters. We reached the finish line elbow to elbow.

The perspective of finishing, the joy of having succeeded to finish the run, the disappearance of fear for ourselves gave us the force needed for this last energetic push.

These 100 km of Millau, it is our life, that's all! The account of these 14 hours of running illustrates the manner in which the body manages its energy potential as a function of trials that are inflicted on it. It tests its capacity to adapt.

- What can we learn from this experience to help maintain good health?

1) Set personal goals in all parts of life.

2) Conceive dreams that are reachable and attain them.

3) Take into account the risks.

4) Advance towards your goals in good humor and share these hopes as much as possible with others.

5) Use the spirit of competition intelligently.

6) Prepare for challenges.

7) Arm oneself with pugnacity and perseverance.

8) Choose the right "tools".

9) Adapt to the situation, the environment in which we live.

10) Know how to modulate, instead of stopping.

11) Self-evaluate and don't renounce at the least alarms

12) Don't confuse tiredness with exhaustion.

13) Listen to alarms. Suffering leads to ruptures. One has to anticipate this, slow down, give the body a chance to rekindle energy for a new project.

14) Don't get exasperated if one feels a total rupture, "a little death". There is always "an afterwards", once energy is reconstituted.

It is not necessary to run the 100km of Millau to understand the conditions of stress that might bring us to a rupture.

They are found inevitably in every life.

There doesn't exist a life without difficulties and therefore efforts. Because paradoxically, it is precisely these efforts that allow us to live again and again.

What doesn't kill you, reinforces you.

9 The neurotherapeutic journey

"Disease is not being sick, but the incapacity to get well."

The neurofunctional diagnosis

- A double diagnosis: organic and neurofunctional

As a doctor, I see myself as making the organic diagnosis which is the most plausible as possible then I translate this into the neurofunctional reality. Next, I establish the neurofunctional diagnosis with respect to the global context.

This means to know how to differentiate in a patient what relates to their organic pathology, their psyche and their neurogenetic status. What is the role played by his neurosis and his pleasure? Everything is important to consider. One can establish a hierarchy of events and even an energetic cost balance. What is the price to pay on the energetic basis for each life event? What is the current impact on life today?

I must know directly what is most important affecting the local or general status of the patient.

- The first encounter: gathering information about the patient

A man of 40 years, tennis player, comes for a consultation because he has elbow pain. Besides this, he declares: "I also have back pain."

"Since when?"

"For some time now."

"Are you in good shape?"

"No, I'm actually a little tired."

I need to be sure sometimes because there can always be a major pathology behind this, so I continue my questioning.

"What is your occupation?"

"I am a businessman."

"Do you have responsibilities?"

"Yes, I manage work parties, sometimes big ones. I deal with customers who are not always easily dealt with. I, I, I..."

I need to understand where the patient is coming from. He doesn't smoke or drink alcohol. I know his family. They are all worthy and quite normal. I also learn that he has sleep problems for some time now. I tell him this:

"Listen to me because the diagnosis is quite simple.

You are exhausted. You are in a small burn-out. Tennis isn't the only reason. At 40 you can't expect to live and play tennis like you did when you were 20. It is naive to think you are not expendable. It is really important what is happening to you. We are going to use these pathological things which are by the way secondary, to give you the capacity to respond to your global condition and try to help you gain insight into your situation..."

In the course of this encounter, I am very thorough: chief complaint, personal medical history, past surgery or medical conditions, the contexts and family history. Are you married or not? Do you have children? Is your family life without problems? Are all your children in good health? How are your parents? Are they elderly? In good health? Has there been a divorce or death in your family?

Finally, I appreciate the financial situation or professional status often carriers of difficulties.

This is how we find the most part pathologies and their cause. The questioning follows a certain logic. All this should be followed up with an examination. Everything like the chief complaint, "My back hurts..." is followed by a life history. "My back has been hurting for 3 days, 3 months, 3 years..."

This doesn't mean revealing any truths to patients but rather to carry out a scientific investigation regrouping the dates when symptoms occurred and comparing them to the dates of simultaneous life events.

Patients find it difficult the first time making the connections. But very quickly, it is they who say, "Yes, I know: it was when my sister told me she had cancer..."

Patients want to attract your attention to their vertebrae, their elbow, their knee. The organic condition that preoccupies them is really only a revealing one. There is never an "isolated" condition. I understand very well that a person with a vertebral fracture will have pain. But what interests me is knowing the severity of the pain and at what rate it will get better. Why does one patient put up with pain and another one does not? From these correlated facts, one can recreate the patients' history and determine the intrinsic components of the pathology in which they are imprisoned.

Neurofunctional history

A mason comes for a consultation with lumbar pain. From what I gather, his back benefits more from his job than it suffers. He did not need to do any weight-training. On the other hand, instead of taking charge of his daily pain and acting in his life to repair successive microtraumatic insults with sessions of neuromedicine (for example!), he just continued putting up with the pain. Moreover, he is overweight and consumes large quantities of alcohol. Fortunately, he doesn't smoke, otherwise, he would have accumulated all the reasons to be exhausted at age 50 years. He complains of sciatica or a discal hernia. If I only treat him for that, he will not have the acute pain, but will not escape chronic pain and exhaustion.

What do I treat? A recent or old history?

One cannot treat a lumbago in a young 20-year-old patient the same way as someone with a long history of pain. In a like manner, you don't have the same disease at 30 years old as if you were 60 and to be sure at 6 years! It is very important to understand, at each age, why there is pain and to treat it accordingly.

We don't all have the same capacity to resolve a similar problem. In reality, each person has a unique proper capability.

Each pathology has its neurofunctional history, which implies making a precise diagnosis that is backed up. Without this diagnosis, a retardation of treatment of a neurofunctional pain can result in a potentially severe organic outcome over time.

All my patients have had illnesses in their past history and they carry these around in the present. They want to remain in their past, forget about the present, and be anxious about the future. To reconcile these patients with their history and to prepare their future is also the role of neuromedicine.

The rolling palpation examination and cartography

First off, we research the patient's pains in order to describe them according to neurologic law. This allows us to link them to a segmental vertebral state (dermatome) and to a central state. To evaluate the level of sensibility, we start by using a very light touch, then we increase in intensity.

The patients tell you where they feel their pain, which they associate with a specific organ. We show them through the rolling palpation that this pain exists over a precise pathway all along the body and that the opposite pathway is indemn of any pain.

This awareness permits the patients to measure a clear decrease in pain after the session (analgesia). Moreover, in the course of further sessions, it permits them to appreciate the improvement in the local state.

We finish by a general rolling palpation over the whole body which eventually reveals unconscious localisations of pain.

We transcribe on a dermatome map the areas of blockage where we are going to carry out especially intense treatment.

After the session of microinjections, we redo the rolling palpation. We find every time an improvement in pain and a relaxing of the subcutaneous muscles.

The choice of the intensity of the treatment

Next is the question of the intensity with which I am going to treat the patient, stimulate them and get them restarted. This will be according to the neurofunctional analysis. I will use an index of intensity to correlate the treated neurologic state and the stimulation I will use. If one strikes under the critical mass threshold of something one wants to change, nothing will happen. We should always strike above this level. However, it is not necessary to strike too hard.

In conventional medicine one puts a big blockbuster in the place where the patient is sick. In neuromedicine, one makes many small microinjections to reach the same result. One discovers quickly that the "big blockbuster" treatment is not an obligation.

The doctor has an idea about the patient, their sensibility and their difficulties. For someone who is afraid the first sessions for example must be carried out with much care. The parents of Romeo, a 4-year-old boy. brought their son to see me for otitis. Actually, his ear was normal, but he had a neurovertebral pain. I questioned Romeo directly: "Listen my little friend, I am going to treat you with a squirt gun, alright?"

"Oh yes, that would be great."

"Here, look! here is how it works…"

And on his skin I squeezed the trigger several times so he got used to the noise.

"You see, it is a squirt gun. Bang! Bang! Now let me get some water for it…"

To treat him, I put in the gun a small needle to the small syringe. I know in no case should this boy feel any injection. The needle hardly even touches the skin, but in a small child this is already an intense stimulation. We have here a hyperactive patient and in doing hardly anything I'm doing a lot.

If I stimulate too much a young girl of 18 years old who suffers from spasmophilia she will have violent reactions. I am going to put her in a stupor for three days. It is not dangerous. But difficult to cope with. It's the same for fragile elderly patients.

So, I modify the intensity of my treatment depending on the patient to treat, through varying the products used, the quantity injected and the number of injection sites.

The treatment scale of my sessions ranges from 1 to 1000. Because to say I inject an infant at 1/10 and adult at 7/10 wouldn't make sense. In general, I inject a young child at 20 and an adult at 500 to 1000. But sometimes just around 50 if I suspect a strong reactivity. The intensity is quite adjustable.

Thus to figure out dosages is the essential element of my work.

Five sessions, 40 Days

- The first session

The first session often goes very well, like it's a gift given to everybody: you take a drug, you go to the chiropractor or osteopath, you have a manipulation done, and it works by the "horizontal pathway" or the pathway of the momentaneous adaptation reserves.

This is the level a drug works at, which by local action decreases the violence of a pathology and fosters development of a general capacity to respond. Here we are in what I call an "atmospheric" situation.

After the first session, if I stop there, I know I leave my patient in his fragile chronic state, because as yet, I have reconstructed nothing. I have merely soothed this patient for the time being without having corrected his real problem. Moreover, it is this treatment of the real problem that allows for re-education to occur.

Each pain deepens its course like a stream. If the cause is severe or if the pain has been present for six months, or one or two years, it has dug out a deep riverbed! Even if you have got the patient up to the riverbank again, they will rapidly fall back to the bottom at the slightest problem in life. And this is what one does treating patients with drugs: "Ah, that was good, they don't feel any more pain." But three months later, they are in pain again.

In neuromedicine one says, "No. I am going to change, modify the frame of the patient and go further." And that is re-education.

- The second session: the entrance to the tunnel

With the second session begins the real treatment.

There was a clearing after the first session, but the patient then enters a sort of reverse funnel. During a cycle of three sessions, or 15 days to one month, the patient will pass through the tube which brings to the flared part of the funnel.

This stage is normal, the aggravation is only temporary.

The tube that I often call "tunnel" overflows little by little and the patient finds a solid ground again, a deep and global adaptation. Not only does the patient no longer feel any pain, but feels more relaxed, less angry.

What happened?

The second session intervened when the patient's latent capacity for adaptation was exhausted. But by the injections, I put the organism back into resistance through recreating a stress. There where I obtained an improvement, I created a crisis. But a very temporary one. I know the body will find its second wind.

I put into motion what I call "the vertical pathway" that gives "turbo" responses to current problems. This opening, the vertical pathway, is a new creation, because your adaptation potential until now was completely disarmed due to exhaustion with age or because of blockage in the young.

- The tunnel

When the patient is in the tunnel, one must maintain confidence in order to peacefully attain the second wind and the opening of the vertical pathway. It is by this pathway that I am creating or recreating the patient's adaptative potential.

For several weeks I have to encourage patients who say: "I'm better, but it's still not right...". They feel depressed, uncomfortable in themselves. They get aggressive with me. They want a cure that they dream about. They had a taste of it at the first session. They feel disappointed and I must keep them going to the end of my wits until about the fifth week.

This period of latency corresponds to a neuroendocrinian phase of maturation and resetting of the nervous centers that manage stress. There is no doubt that this involves a process of general cerebral adaptation, and not a local reaction over the pathways and the site of pain.

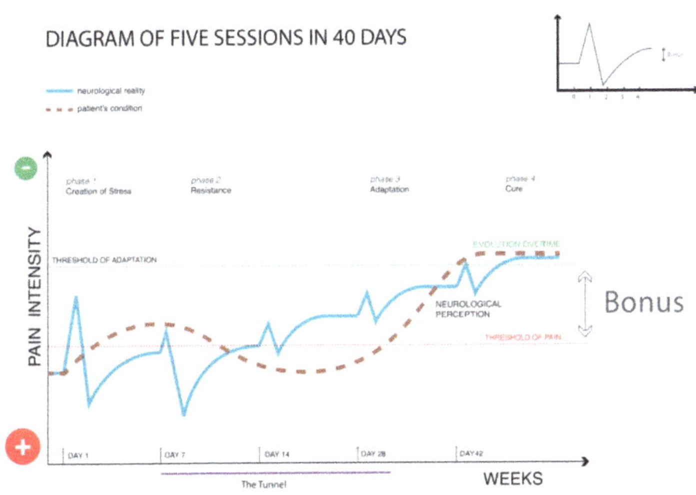

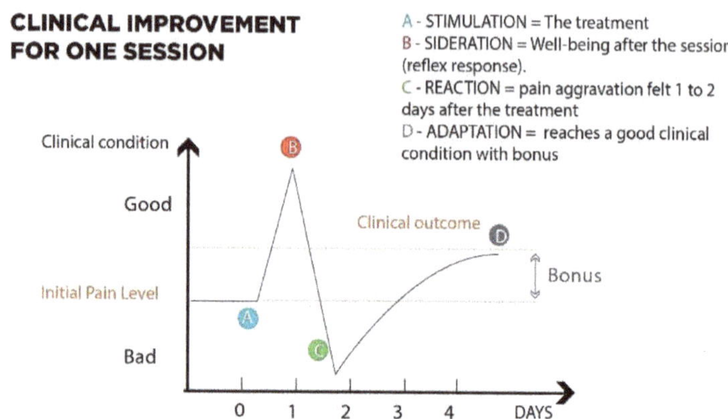

At the exit of the tunnel, the patient will have had five sessions. The organism will have been treated five times in a row and will have by this fact completed the journey of care: this journey of calling into question, of reconstruction of a durable, solid response capable of protecting the patient lastingly. The fifth session comes in order to reinforce the acquired state.

The complete cycle of a lasting transformation will have taken 40 days

- Reconstruction

Neuromedicine invites patients to re-explore, relive what they knew how to do before but that they had completely lost the habit of doing. They always took the easy way out by doing what they could still do "Because I can do it, I know I am not ill!" – until they got exhausted and lost the capacity of a healthy, realistic response.

Patients are reborn, with an ability to adapt incomparable to their previous life. This was not just out of addressing myself to the problem the patient came for, knee pain or digestive problem. But also with regard to their global past. They will be ten times less anxious and much less tired now. They might even be able to make decisions like: "I will lose weight", "I'm starting gym again", "I am going to be different with my entourage", "I am going to quit smoking.

Patients are now capable of leaving behind their old life where they were stuck, and which through escape or un-willingness led them, little by little, to a failure, at least in the domain of their health.

Contrary to a drug, which leads to a failure because it maintains you in "a state", neuromedicine can give you a new outlook of yourself, and not that which you had prior to illness. But that of "you in perspective" of a real adap-tation potential and thus a change. A rebirth of sorts.

10 Exemplary case reports

"To treat pain is possible for everyone, but going further than the pain is not."

We have chosen some case histories for which neuromedicine seems to be able to give new answers to. We would also like to emphasize the common points that exist among them.

Acute cases, chronic cases

In neuromedicine we systematically link the organ involved with the nerve centers of the spinal cord (segmentary level). For the calf, the regulatory zones are located at the bottom of the spinal cord where the roots L3-S3 arise. DIAGR M. They involve the controls of sensibility, motor function, muscle tone, etc...

The supra-segmentary level (medulla oblongata and hypothalamus) comprises two parts: one specific, in charge of the local problem and one non-specific which manages stress and intervenes globally on survival functions. In a first phase, these two responses complement each other.

- Sprain: caring for an acute injury.

If this is a benign ankle sprain, the patient first feels a sharp pain, then is unable to walk. The radiographic film shows nothing. A partial rupture of the external lateral ligament nevertheless provoked an immediate bleeding. A "pigeon's egg" is formed. One must therefore immobilise the foot so that the ligament can heal.

Some patients go see the chiropractor who manipulates the ankle saying, "I'm putting it back in place." When one leaves the chiropractor, one suffers less due to the analgesic effect created by the nerve centers of the spinal cord. By adding a stress to a stress, the doctor reactivated the "gate control" and started instantly a neurologic stable inhibition of the pain, the inflammation and the cramps.

In neuromedicine we add a general stimulation to the local treatment by injections over the sensitive cutaneous zones which we find by rolling palpation. These zones we find all the way to the buttock (segmentary level) to the neck (supra-segmentary level).

The injections add a medullary stress to the acutely affected ligament and its neurologic consequences thus triggering deblocking phenomenas at the segmentary and suprasegmentary levels.

The edema is greatly reduced in two or three days.

The delay of recovery using a conventional cast is from 20 to 45 days and often with 3 months of rehabilitation. Using neuromedicine allows a more rapid recovery.

I treat sprains without fracture but ligament damage in 45 days without a cast – muscles will not undergo wasting – and no rehabilitation. The patient walks without a crutch in ten days but with a support stocking. Some sessions of physiotherapy help out.

Contrary to the efficient action of the chiropractor, which is limited to the local dimension, neuromedicine puts back the lesion and its resolution into the hands of the global nervous system. The patient avoids in this way opportunistic interactions such as fatigue, mood disorders. The follow-up also reduces the risk of chronic pain.

- Sprain: caring for a chronic case.

Mr. C, 50 years old, is tired by his work. He doesn't get much exercise. He is overweight and smokes. He is living thus on his reserves. One day, he sprains his ankle skiing. He comes in to see me three months later with ankle pain which prevents him from walking despite physical therapy and drugs.

He has created a neurofunctional disease in a deficient state. The minor ligamentary affection repaired itself in 20 days, but the pain is still there. Why? The sprain led to an overcharge of his state of fatigue and put him into a situation of unadapted excessive response.

Rolling palpation finds evidence of pain along the L5 dermatome. However, his exhausted nervous system does not react strongly as in the case of an acute sprain. Only a complete "40 day session with 5 stimulations" can allow him local relief and to treat his state of exhaustion.

Pre-operatory and post-operatory

One should consider each operation as an insult and most particularly for those exhausted patients. Operatory shocks should be preceded by neuromedicine to prepare the nervous system around the affected organ which will be operated on. Without this precaution, complications such as pain or infection occur more frequently. For example, I don't think that we should ever operate a person over 20 with a painful knee if it is accompanied by exhaustion. A minimum amount of recovery of adaptation is needed first.

Mrs. W came to see me about sharp knee pain that persisted after surgery for two months. She was among the 80 % of patients however which should normally have recovered in this time by developing good adaptation responses. This inadaptation struck me as surprising, but I understood why when she told me that she had been operated on several days after the death of her mother. A patient in mourning should be taken into account. One must not do surgery in this context.

I propose to her 5 sessions over 40 days to resolve this double problem: that of the mourning and that of the post-op knee pain. This problem once well-diagnosed and treated, was resolved.

I often intervene in post-operatory pain, edema, cramps in patients who can't seem to recover quickly. Often one single session is enough.

There should be a Department of neuromedicine in every hospital like there is a Department of Intensive Care.

The particular case of neurogenic pain

Mrs. G, 68 years old, has chronic back pain. Three years back these pains only appeared on effort or at the end of the day. For a little while now, they have become constant with bursts that she can't take anymore and for which drugs proved ineffective. Imagery of her spinal column showed nothing. Neither are there any digestive problems that could cause transferred pain.

She is weakened psychologically by her pains, and she talks very emotionally about them, holding back her tears. She has so wrestled with this state that she is now in what I call a kind of chronic exhaustion, a "depression of the body".

These neurogenic pains slowly became chronic. They are not from a local disorder but translate a neurologic pathology which has become structural and global in nature.

The reactions to rolling palpation are so prominent that one has the impression that there is an "emotional wound" under our fingers that gives a concrete reality of pain to the patient whom can finally be seen and recognised.

Contrary to the current theory, neurogenic pains do not seem to me to be limited to the destruction or lesions of a peripheral or central nerve structure, but to be associated with a deep dysfunctioning of "pain" function.

The pain is felt locally, then circulates according to different loops between the site of pain and the places where it is perceived: the nervous centers of the spinal column and the brain. The neuronal influx that carries this pain is usually modulated even inhibited, but in this case there is no regulation at all.

In the pain Centers, despite their quality treatment, conventional theory reaches its limits. In effect, these pains are resistant to many drugs and other treatments.

Here, neuromedicine can show it's great usefulness. Neurological re-education finishes by controlling these pains if enough time is allowed and if preconceived notions about organ-centered pains are modified.

Most cases of neurogenic pain are resolved in 40 days. This was the case for Mr. V who was an amputee of both legs above the knee suffering from phantom pains. Over the last 20 years, his rare relapses of pain were cured within one session.

More difficult cases require much longer treatment times, sometimes over years.

Back Pain

Back pain causes the most absences from work in France. Most manual workers think that the physical labor they do at work is enough to maintain them in good condition. This is a big mistake. Even if their job allowed them to get a good musculature. At the same time they are working, the repetition of movements has led to a localised chronic suffering where arthritis lurks about.

More than other folks, they need to have a physical activity which is vigorous over a short time, thus inhibiting any functional lesions of their back from working daily. Because they don't, a durable body debt occurs. And inevitably, they have back pain.

This is also true for those persons who do not have a manual job. In fact, as it is now, 80 % of back pain is attributed to vertebral lesions or arthritis and 20 % to lifestyle. In reality it is the opposite. Treatment by neuromedicine in this domain has few failures. Rolling palpation demonstrates that the entire spine is involved, not just the site of the pain. This pathology is due to a neurofunctional exhaustion and translates the inadaptation: "I get back pain because I am surrounded by work and I am tired for quite a while now."

Neuromedicine does not just treat the pain, like a drug does. It is interested in the reason for the pain and rehabilitates the regulatory circuits of energy. Rolling palpation at all levels shows if the recovery is complete or partial regardless of what the patient feels. This prevents vertebral aging and relapses.

Fibromyalgia and burn-out

Fibromyalgia cannot be defined as a somatic state because there are often no causes found for the pain or insignificant rheumatological ones. It is also not a depression. But all patients with it complain of tiredness.

If it is not somatic or mental, then what is it? These are states of neurologic exhaustion, the reason for the existence of neuromedicine.

Surely one must agree that fibromyalgia is very complex. Moreover, the exhaustion affects the management of pain and energy but also willpower: the ability to make decisions decreases.

There is a questionable doubt in medical circles on the existence of this disease recently recognised. Organic causes are incriminated abusively because this is reassuring. Often the muscles are held responsible, there must be a guilty party...

This doubt reinforces my theories on neurofunctional disease. Fibromyalgia exists for sure with its cortège of diffuse pain and inflammation. Roughly 80% of the patients are hyperactive women who never quit and who wrestled too much...

I associate fibromyalgia with "burn-out". This latter is to acute forms what fibromyalgia is to chronic forms. A dozen years separates the two states.

To treat fibromyalgia or burn-out is to treat neurologic exhaustion. The little injections work miracles with the progressive abolition of pain and the reconstitution of an adaptive potential to stress. In living organisms, all improvement in results of disease, affects it's cause. So, it is here also and there is hope.

Addiction is innate in humans

All my patients are addicts. You eat too much? Even if it isn't understood as that: you are an addict. You love children too much? You are an addict. You love your work too much? You are an addict. This full-up of "whatever " puts us in an obsessional vortex that exhausts us and winds up creating an energy vacuum, this void causes a rupture and the breach creates the disease.

Disease is to have done the same thing too much, to get saturated. Patients come because they have a complaint, not necessary to resolve the cause of it. They come because they have pain. And when we have pain we go see the doctor. "I caught cold, I have bronchitis. I've been putting up with it for a week". I know, he knows that after three days it isn't a sufficient reason. The truth is he smokes a lot and the tobacco created an immune deficit and local inflammation by neurologic exhaustion. The slightest fatigue can be a decompensatory factor towards infection in the smoker. He could have also said: "Since I am angry with my neighbor, I can't stop coughing." Every "conflict" will add on to the tobacco stress in him.

What is true for smoking is also true for other addictions.

I don't know how to oblige anyone to stop smoking or stop drinking. But if I lead him into this process and he does it, I can accompany him. I know how to treat withdrawal syndromes for bulimia and poorly contained states of aggressivity. The response to the stress of the injections is durable for withdrawal and makes it much more palatable. The period of injections is 40 days, 5 sessions. Failure is very rare.

There does exist severe addictive states where neuromedicine doesn't work, since the point of no return has been reached. However, I treated patients on substitution drugs for opiate addiction and helped them recover their emotional stability more quickly. This helped them to return to a satisfactory social life.

It's difficult for a doctor to accept that our life could be deprecated for a few sublime pleasures, soon to be duds compared to the usual highs and lows of our lives, maintaining our spring.

Overweightness and obesity

- Overweightness

People who have this problem are very aware of it. To be socially accepted is often an indispensable alternative for living. Overweightness is a symptom that results from several problems often old ones. It has for a cause excessive overeating which is especially self-regulated until a stable weight is reached. But this weight is often unsatisfactory.

Neuromedicine treats overweightness at several levels:

1) at the global level by decreasing fatigue and stress induced by the increased awareness and a better hygiene in life;

2) at the local level by stopping excitability of digestive zones as found on rolling palpation. To remove the blockages generally causes bulimia to disappear. Moreover, for women, the treatment allows a reduction in cellulitis and its harmful local effects (subcutaneous inflammation) which affects the general condition.

- Obesity

Obesity is a severe neurofunctional state which needs to be approached as certain dependant addictive states, but also is a behavioural disorder. One is not cured by good advice or by force. These patients have an insatiable appetite so their solution can only be found in turning to food. Any retardation only exacerbates this feeling of absolute need where neurosis and guilt are added. Curing it is uncertain because the profusion of energy englobes the body and spirit in a point of no return.

The neurologic tension involved is so high that willpower is neutralised.

Nevertheless, neuromedicine can decrease stress, the consequences of hepatic steatosis from bulimia, and fatigue.

Aging

Aging is a natural phenomenon that has a limit in time, but also gives to our lives a sense and value. I don't think we can modify this time limit, except maybe fiddle with genes to retard the programming.

Throughout our life our bereavements, our pains, our trials accumulate in an unconscious way. Tiredness, pain, diseases become more and more severe, adding to the distress.

In the long term, these overloads pile up. Combined with our genetic heritage they create a "trunk", becoming heavier and heavier to carry around. Without any preparation for aging the global adaptation potential decreases and every event provokes exacerbated reactions that self-generate.

Neuromedicine has a role to play to accompany aging. It allows renegotiation of the weight of the "trunk".

With age, it is no longer a question of performance but landing smoothly. To have pain is maybe a chance... One can build up from this pain which renders one conscious of life. How can we get out of this vicious circle of pain and disease to give us some pleasant years of life before term? How can we act to preserve our health?

Elderly patients in pain that come to see me ever y two months have a completely different quality of life. I plaster up the insults in their lives. Without pretense of curing disease and even less of preventing death, I simply try to create adaptation potential.

Through its stimulations in response to pain, neuromedicine fills the absence of any "stressful" activity which is so needful at this age. The repeated demands through the treatment on the nervous system leads the patient to develop a response that can be classified as a resistance. And this neurologic resistance is really the only preventive treatment for aging. Resistance to temptations to overeat, to be idle, to let things go, to be complacent in front of sadness or frustrations. Quite simply: pain resistance.

My medical center is a nursery of hundred-year-olds!

Thirty years ago we spoke little of this disease as we ascribed it to senile dementia.

However, as early as 1906, Dr. Alzheimer asked himself about its origin because he had a fifty-year-old patient with it.

Very specific cerebral lesions in this dementia lead to the gradual loss of cognitive functions like memory. Life no longer belongs to the patient but to his body only dedicated to his survival but penalised by a constant and reactional stress.

Here we have a neurologic degradation that I attribute in part or all to a failure of neurological centers, i.e. a hyperactive state of a deregulated neurologic function.

If we make an exception of the cases that affect young patients, Alzheimer's disease is a disease of aging whose increase yearly is 5% after age 80.

An early treatment as possible is best, even before onset. At age 60 years, people should go to see a neuromedical doctor for preventive treatment. Inevitably, rolling palpation detects pathways of neurogenic pain, which intervenes in aging and Alzheimer's disease.

Furthermore, hygienic measures will permit the establishment of more well-balanced neurologic circuits: eating, exercise, intellectual and emotional life. Thus, athletes are affected by senile dementia up to 50% less frequently. Their actions are a testimony to the preventive effect of neurologic stimulations.

Cancer

Cancer is a disease of neurologic exhaustion in a chain re-action. When the cells no longer accept their conditions and when the neurologic circuits become incoherent.

We don't treat cancer with neuromedicine. However, as in all domains of medicine, neuromedicine has uses in two areas: prevention and postcure.

- Prevention

Mastosis is the origin of many breast cancers. This is a chronic inflammatory state of the mammary glands that affects one woman in two to various degrees. The classic treatment is with progesterone. In most cases they soothe the painful stages, but the inflammation remains.

A follow-up in the long run by neuromedicine allows sig-nificant reduction of inflammation and edema. In this way it slows down the potential occurrence of cancer in women who are calmed and aware of the risk.

This specific prevention can be applied to other types of cancer notably prostate or colon cancer.

Furthermore, all neurofunctional treatment has a global preventive effect because it provides again energy for pa-tients who adopt a good hygiene in life: reasonable eating habits, practicing a sport on a regular basis. Thus we know that among athletes again, the incidence of cancer is two-fold less than in the general population.

Mr. B is treated for leukemia. His drug therapy is a real trial for him. His body seems strange and he can't stand anything. He has hemorrhoids, which add to his misery from the pain. He feels next to an abyss.

The rolling palpation is without surprise. It instantly reveals the neuralgic circuits and their contacts up to the neck and down to the ankle on the left-hand side. His exacerbated state under these circumstances of major neurologic stress calls for very delicate stimulations. But rolling palpation permits to see an immediate cutaneous impact. From the day after the session, an improvement is seen, which is confirmed in the following days.

Not long later, the suffering was displaced to the right where hepatic toxicity caused by the drugs caused nausea and pain.

The neuromedical treatment yields partial sedation which is encouraging. In the long run, drug cures are better tolerated. Reactions become more tolerable and, of course, are shorter. It goes without saying that this is an effective treatment and a comforting one in times of trial.

So there exists a common key in all these pathologies. Whatever they are, the patient is confronted with a major neurologic medullary reaction which is added to the disease.

They could have been treated before their appearance, which if it didn't prevent the disease it would slow it up.

Once the pathology takes hold, the patient's body fights the disease, causing stress. They can benefit from treatment in postcure to smooth over the secondary effects of drugs and attenuate the intensity of their fight.

Thus, neuromedicine will not treat a heart attack, but can complement preventive measures. If it does happen however, it can treat in postcure the myocardiopathies, frequent neurological complications which occur.

One can ask the question: is there just one disease?

No, but the nervous system intervenes in all pathologies. It always adds a neurofunctional disease to the organic one.

11 Placebo et Nocebo

"Placebo + Nocebo = Turbo"

Placebo

- What is a Placebo?

Placebo effect is an improvement in the disease felt by a patient who took a "drug" that contained no active ingredient for which it was prescribed.

Furthermore, above drug-taking, any treatment having no effective action on a recognized pathology but that is nevertheless followed by a positive effect, we can call a placebo. This principle can be applied in a like manner to the intervention of a health care deliverer no matter what the nature.

We attribute this to the positive attitude of a consented upon medical procedure.

The kings of France put their hands on scrofula (cutaneous tuberculous lesions) to cure it. Among animists, the witch doctor cures by words that transcend evils. After some incantations, he exclaims: "Go home, you are cured!" This is inscribed in individuals of the same culture and unifies them. He confers on the sick a capacity to be cured multiplied by the confidence in his powers. The sick person can only be comforted more by the addition of a herbal drug known from ancestral times.

The most important force behind the placebo effect is surely the doctor himself. This is the decisive factor in triggering the placebo effect in the patient. It has been shown that a doctor's receptiveness, an empathetic attitude, attentive explanations, multiply the placebo effect.

One could conceive of no better placebo than a Medical School Professor. Thanks to renowned competency, the doctor has the highest amount of credibility, and one has blind faith (but merited in this case) in the professor's capability.

This "power" uses pathways that remain to this day largely misunderstood.

Several explanations have been proposed. The first is psychological. Some researchers evoke suggestiveness. For others, placebo effect is a conditioned reflex.

The hypothesis which I like can well compliment the aforementioned ones. It involves neurobiological mechanisms. Endorphins, endogenous morphines secreted by the nervous system at the hypothalamus level, act to decrease pain. Their liberation is due to the positive feeling of the patient who proceeds to consult the doctor. It is like a neurologic bonus of hope. Other neuromediators like dopamine favor at the same time a feeling of well-being.

All diseases don't respond to placebo and all patients nether. Functional pathologies like painful states, headaches or digestive problems respond better to placebo than organic conditions with a lesion.

In neuromedicine, we consider that functional betterment aids organic betterment and that the placebo also acts on many minor organic conditions.

Placebo effect is seen among non-scientific persons in a pejorative way. It is seen as a mystical effect. Patients that respond positively to a placebo are taken for simpletons or gullible persons. This is an error.

Moreover, the effectiveness of placebo drugs has been proven in double-blind drug trials as compared to drugs with an active ingredient.

- Placebo in neuromedicine

Like all therapies neuromedicine has a placebo dimension. It is important to dwell on this for two reasons: 1) to respond to the negative connotation of placebo which seems to be given to all non-conventional medical practices; and 2) because it is possible that the mode of action of neuromedicine is that of placebo amplified by the stimulations that exacerbate the response.

Disease puts our body in tension. It is testimony of a conflict in our organism, the latter which tends to maintain homeostasis at all costs. This means the permanent maintenance of an internal balance with regard to incessant variations of the external world.

As we have seen already, the sudden stimulation of the injections creates a stress, which adds to the demands made by the disease state. In this rapid and systematic reaction placebo and psychology play no role.

It is after this purely neurologic step that the placebo effect is ever-present when the patient undergoes a treatment in which he believes will work.

In decreasing all the tensions by a rebound effect like a "tsunami" of endorphins, it potentializes the neurologic response in a positive direction. The induced "placebo" becomes "turbo". This effect or "placeturbo" unlike placebo, can be triggered voluntarily. Putting the organism in danger induces a positive response.

Doctor Nocebo

Placebo: I am liked. Nocebo: I am not liked. The Nocebo is one of the preponderant actors of neuromedicine.

The stronger I inject strongly, the more I insist, the more I put the organism in jeopardy, the more my patient reacts doubts: I am nocebo, I am not liked. "This doctor is "killing" me. He hurts me. It's taking a long time..."

As we have seen, in acute states during two days the specific exacerbated reaction caused by neuromedicine results in a lethargy. In the course of the forty days crossing the desert, the pathology comes back in a latent and silent way. The pains that persist play a nocebo role. Still felt, they appear locally as "burst". They act in the sense of the Nocebo.

Paradoxically, and especially concerning the negative aspect, the reaction yet induces a powerful neurologic stress. The negative exaggeration created by the injections accompanied by the instant reaction of rejection by the patient, potentializes in the long term an exponential positive response of survival. This response elicited goes against disease factors. It reinforces and liberates the process of adaptation which leads to a cure.

The response at the first session of Mrs. D, 65 years old, was very positive. But at the second session she broke down and wept... "I came 100 miles to see you and it doesn't work!" The relapse after an initial improvement is felt as a bereavement. So why did she come back?

Instead of keeping away from the Doctor Nocebo that I have become in her eyes, due to the aggravation, she felt comforted by my treatment. She was given a warning. She no longer was herself. An active response was occurring in her nerve centers. Mrs. D's case follows the reactive principles of her treatment even if her words suggest the contrary. She was no longer capable of quitting because the work going on in her body was monopolizing all her energy. She improved slowly until she had no pain but it came unawares in successive steps until she was cured.

One can suggest here that a process of maturation took place like a state of self-hypnosis. It is like if I had enclosed her in this reaction which leads her at its end to a liberation and thus a cure.

Placebo and Nocebo act together. One is positive and the other negative. Placebo inhibits disease by liberation of neuromediators. But Nocebo, through exaggeration, amplifies survival reflexes. In the end it plays a positive role like placebo.

12 Where it is a question of failure

"It's going to turn out poorly. The way is therefore important."

As I have explained in the previous chapters, I am convinced that my therapeutic procedure can benefit 100 % of patients for the treatment of chronic diseases or as an adjunct therapy in severe illnesses.

Nevertheless, I must admit that I don't always get the results I aim for.

The following cases delineate the limits, the obstacles that neuromedicine encounters.

The limits of the therapist: the disease comes first

I tried to treat Mrs. X. I knew that she had been under treatment for a bipolar disorder. But I think that these conditions are quite responsive to the therapy I offer.

After two or three sessions, she disclosed to me her difficulties, her relapses and her neurotic states.

And I understood that she was in fact in an equilibrium with her pathology. To cure this woman neuromedicine would just strongly upset this equilibrium. So I found it prudent to stop treatment. I didn't feel comfortable with taking the risk of destabilizing her, of recreating a severe psychotic episode. To help her recover her tranquility, I offered to remain her therapist. I wanted to imply that she could recover. I let her leave with this in mind, that there must be a way.

When the patient is the beneficiary of his disease

I am sometimes confronted with patients who don't want to lose their authority. In this, I mean that they want to be well, but not to face any changes. They remain for the time being beneficiaries of their pathology.

Mrs. J came for a consultation because she had a new episode of sharp chronic lumbar pain. I see her two or three times in the month before finding an improvement in rolling palpation. She denies getting any better. I learn that this 75-year-old lady lives alone. Her daughter lives 30 miles away. Since her mother has been ill, she has been coming to see her once or twice a week bringing her food and doing some of her housework. The daughter never did this before. I conclude that Mrs. J prefers to be ill and thus see her daughter.

Mr. Y has had chronic gonalgia for years. He lives 80 miles from the medical center. When he comes, he uses the occasion to visit a friend. After the first session, I suggest coming back in a month which he accepts. The day before the session he calls me to cancel it. "Your session really helped me, but I have to be re-examined by the Health Authority about my disability benefits. I'm afraid of being too well and then they would decrease my benefits."

When entourage is beneficiary of the disease

Mrs. F felt so ill that I had to make a home visit to treat her. I had had positive results in the past concerning her pain. But now it didn't work anymore. One day her husband, exasperated to see me, interjected: "When do you count on curing her? It sure is taking a long time". And I retorted, "My dear sir, when you cease to bring back all these bottles home that I can see piled up under the sink she might have a chance to get better."

The husband bought his peace of mind by keeping his wife in her dependence on alcohol.

Submission to conventional medicine

Mr. D is a 60-year-old capable cross-country runner who can run a marathon under 3 hours. He comes to consult because he has pain after an excessive effort. But it is his last resort. I know he saw another doctor, took drugs, and consulted an osteopath. Nothing worked!

He expects me to treat him for his acute problem out of despair, but he doesn't consider me his therapist in the long run for his general problems. He reserves that for the conventional doctor.

In this case, the limits of neuromedicine are inherent in the role assigned to the doctor by the patient. So then the role of the neuromedical doctor is to explain ways to resolve the problem, for cure, without being overbearing. The idea working its way in may be sufficient to induce a positive reaction.

Mrs. H has sciatica for two months. On examination of her hip, it was not particularly painful. Through rolling palpation I get directly to diagnosis.

"It is a cruralgia."

Then with a furious look, she interrupts me: "How can you say that? My doctor told me I have sciatica!"

"Did your doctor examine you undressed?"

"No. He had me do a scan."

So I look at the images which effectively show a mild lower lumbar discal pinching which could provoke a sciatica. But in this case the pathway of pain is absolutely not that of sciatica, but that of a cruralgia.

Her doctor did not examine her hip, her knees or the spine. His diagnosis is definitely mistaken. In conventional medicine whether it is sciatica or cruralgia doesn't change the treatment. One prescribes A.I.N.S. drugs.

But in re-educative medicine, I need to differentiate between the two so I can apply an appropriate treatment to cure the patient.

Mrs. H cannot accept this treatment if she does not believe in my diagnosis. If she doesn't extricate herself from this blind medicine, it will be difficult for me to help her.

Patient inability to go beyond his local problem

I treated Mr. S four or five years ago for his back pain. During the time he didn't see me he gained 40-50lbs. This time he has left shoulder pain. On examining his images and his shoulder, his shoulder is not the problem.

Mr. S is in a state of exhaustion. I could not get him to divulge the circumstances which made him put on so much weight.

In this case, I haven't any room to maneuver, because the patient is consulting ONLY for this pain. Whatever my efforts may be, as long as I can't learn the global picture, the resolution will only be a partial one. He is incapable of telling me his life events which could help me orient his treatment, I am simply going to relieve his shoulder pain, but nothing else.

Natural limits

Mr. M, 60 years old, was brought to me by his wife for his back pain. He also suffered from respiratory failure putting in question his vital prognosis. He was literally out of breath. His wife incessantly repeated to me: "Tell him to walk. He doesn't listen to me. He must do some walking."

At this stage, re-education through physical activity was too late. I could relieve his back pain, but I could not give him enough power to move forward. The insistence of his wife just complicated things.

So I turned to her and said: "Madame, your husband can no longer walk, but at least you could love him..."

Medicines of re-education can only work when there is an ability to react. We treat life with life.

In some situations, one cannot any longer expect to improve. Either because advanced age does not allow it or because the equilibrium of the situation must not be disturbed. Improvement would almost be dangerous because it would derange the global equilibrium.

Now this does not mean there is nothing we can do. The problem is to accompany these patients. The goal is to respect the clinical reality of the patient avoiding any ruptures which could occur if the therapeutic program was poorly explained and if unfounded hopes were suggested.

13 The psychological dimension

"A conventional doctor is sure of his drug but I am sure of my patient."

In neuromedicine, treatment of a disease always takes the corresponding underlying affective psychological dimension into account. It uses it as an additional lever to allow healing to take place in a global physical, psychological and neurologic dimension.

The triggering event

In his book "The Theory of Somatic Markers" previously mentioned, Antonio Damasio considers that we are "body-soul" entities. Emotions stem from the mind but they only exist through body expression. The body serves as a vase of expansion. We think that the neurologic circuits he mentions are precise and identifiable by rolling palpation.

The somatic manifestation of emotions is resorbed spontaneously over variable period of time. If this does not occur, this emotional state endures and disease occurs. The appearance of a symptom in acute disorders or an exacerbation in a chronic condition is explained by an emotional trauma. In acute conditions, it is the intensity that induces blockage, while in chronic states it is the phenomenon of accumulation.

The individual response to this event is unique for each patient and neither proportional to the severity nor the nature of the cause.

This fact is collectively denied by the medical milieu trained only to see an organic problem. And also by the patients themselves out of fear of the intangible in their eyes.

The relationship of the doctor with the patient is thus essential. A verbal exchange reveals the triggering event and helps to understand the environment in which it is expressed.

A young woman comes for a consultation because she has stomachache for three days. I reveal to her that three days ago she had scolded her granddaughter and locked her up in her bedroom. She was worried not to hear her granddaughter, so she opened the bedroom door. She noticed the child had pooped on the floor rug. The reaction of her daughter convinced her that she had acted too harshly. Her guilt triggered in her an acid stomach.

Mrs. X says to me she has a pain for 6 months. When I asked her what had happened in her life 6 months ago she couldn't really say. 8 days later in a new consultation, she said now she remembered that 6 months ago she had learned her son was getting a divorce.

One of my patients had sciatica at about the same time every year. There was never any explanation found for this in a CT-scan. She finally realised that this pathology coincided with the anniversary of her father's death.

A patient was really involved in the organisation of a public event in which he would give a speech. The night before the event, he felt intense hip pain and discovered later he had coxarthrosis. I helped him realise that he had not resolved the causes of his great bashfulness.

Mrs. G, 50 years old and administrative secretary, had back pain for two months and incriminated arthritis as the cause. She finally understood that it was at work that she created this problem. She trained a colleague in her job to help out and the colleague took her job. She was transferred to a remote place.

These examples are not just a few particular cases. For each one of us, our daily emotional life is involved in say a wry neck, a fatigue, an anger, an arthritis of the knee that starts to be a pain. The presence of this peripheral pain reveals this to us and prevents us from advancing forward.

Resolution

The patient does the work, I never replace them because it is through their reaction that they find their cure. As their past weigh down their present so much, I am there to help them before and after.

I help them arrange their room, reconcile with themselves, and to break away.

Arrange his room.

"What do you mean arrange my room?"

"You have played with this, then that, and that. Only you have never arranged things for many years. You navigate daily in this too-full of junk room so it is tiring. However, you can't help yourself. To change your state of things you need energy which you don't have. You're exhausted. It's time to put things in order, to reorganise your existence and to re-establish a reasonable hierarchy of your priorities."

A woman who had gone on a three-week holiday in the sun came to consult me as soon as she returned.

"What brings you in? I asked her."

"During my three-week holiday I had absolutely no pain. But as soon as I walked in the door of my house I had back pain! How can you explain that, doctor?"

It was quite easy for me to explain why. She returned to "her room" in the same state as when she left it before this period of rest and relaxation.

Reconcile patients with themselves

Through rolling palpation, I detect zones of suffering in my patients. These are a testimony to the conflicts in their body. Some are old and unresolved, maintaining them in an enduring energy deficit. A new conflict, even a mild one, sets off the powder keg.

How can we claim to cure a patient when we can't get them to reconcile with themselves? How can we help them make their way towards a greater maturity? Neuromedicine through its re-education of nerve centers, renders them competent and capable of self-evaluation.

Mr. D, slightly obese, consulted for a pain between the shoulder blades. The cycle of five sessions allowed him to resolve the problem. His increased mobility and my encouragements incited him to take up a physical activity. He lost weight. Little by little he slipped out of a state of conflict to a state of self-confidence. This gave him the possibility to live in a guilt-free present and to make plans for a realistic future. I recommended that he not fall back into the old lifestyle, which would cause a relapse.

Victor, a 17-year-old, came to consult me for an Osgood-Schlatter Disease or a painful inflammation of the knee which appeared when he was growing up. His age indicated to me that this diagnosis was improbable. I tried to cure him in 40 days but after more than 80 days I had not succeeded in relieving his pain completely.

His images showed nothing so I could set aside the somatic problem in favor of a psychological one.

Why did this boy get ill? The boy's mother was always present during the consultations. The boy let his mother do all the talking for him, however, he was old enough to do the talking himself as a future adult.

My role was to give time to allow Victor to realise it was his problem. The pain decreased and the symptom was played down which put into doubt the somatic reality. Through my advice, I meanwhile instilled another possible scenario for the mother-son relationship.

We can well see in this case how neuromedicine radically goes beyond the local field to take on the psychological reality of this young man.

Mr. S is too fat and he knows it. He is a man who lives alone and "in overindulgence". He consults me for a shoulder pain, but it is evident that his global problem is more important than the local one. He is a man who has been in conflict for too long and he is more than just exhausted. One must not push him in the wrong direction which would make him feel guilty. So first I prefer to relieve his pain. The physical improvement that he feels is a link between us. Afterward I will see what he does with it... Sometimes even years later.

Mrs. G's husband is waiting for her in the waiting room. When the session is too long, I can tell he gets impatient. I have no doubt that this husband is a fact involved in her neurosis.

At the end of six months, she is much better. And without any psychological input on my part. I'm sure she has marital problems, but I never said anything to her. Nevertheless, I did say to her: "Mrs. G, you know through these injections, we have created an adaptation potential. Your suffering deprived you of defending yourself. Don't use this newfound capability to submit to more problems."

Without specifically delineating the problems, this suggestive discussion almost always hits the bull's eye. Patients recognize themselves. I give them keys to take their life in hand without creating new conflicts with others.

It is not about denouncing their lifestyle (that is out of the question) but helping them to live better, feeling serene, learning the expression of happy ideas.

My patients are not ill enough psychologically to need a psychotherapist. I can advise them. For some – they are usually between 35 and 50 years old – I suggest doing some psychotherapeutic sessions as well because I know they would benefit from it and reap a rapid profit out of sorting out complicated situations. For the others, the work we do together gives them the time to evolve at their own speed.

Their pain, their behavior, or whoever it is in their entourage should not serve as a justification or an alibi.

My role is to make them freer and more capable in the end: "You don't belong to anyone! Not even your work or your spouse and even less your children!"

We all have a self that needs defining, and your liberty belongs only to you.

Present day medicine is focused on organicity and too rarely considers the psychological aspect of illnesses. For neuromedicine, it is essential to use a pain as a potential for stimulation.

I go further than empathy for my patient. I look for the sudden or latent causes of psychological disorders which led to disease. As soon as the patient has identified its causes, psychotherapeutic work begins.

This is not really official psychotherapeutic sessions, but a start which, with time, contributes to a cure.

14 The ways to a cure

"Let your shadow catch up to you"

A cure in spite of you

For his third session, I made Mr. S wait and when I went to call him in, he rushed out of the waiting room like a mad man and literally accosted me.

He said, "This is doing nothing! I ask myself what I am doing here! It's a waste of time! I have better things to do than to have myself treated by people incapable of curing me!"

He was so negative I had nothing to lose. I made myself a mirror to him. I hit him with some reflections about his lifestyle and to finish off, I asked him, "Good, and now can we resume work?"

He followed me into the treatment room.

Mr. S was in "the tunnel" full of doubts. This outburst against me showed especially that he displaced the problem, that he refused to admit that his lifestyle was in large part responsible for his disease.

You are ill because you have exceeded your adaptation capacity. For a long time you have been making an unconscious decision to be ill. Because you ignored the minor warning symptoms.

You come to buy some treatment with a limited view of the causes of your illness and a linear conception of your eventual route to a cure.

Neuromedicine will trigger a process towards a cure that will be opposite to your chosen current lifestyle and thus contrary to you. To reach its goals, the neuromedical doctor intervenes in many ways: intensity and localization of the stimulations, nature and dilution of the products used, and handling of the patient.

It is, however, difficult to know at what time a neurologic threshold will be reached whereby a cure is in play. In fact, in re-education, the organism determines the result: it reacts when it can and is cured... if it wants this. Only a problem of time.

To accept to be better

The first time that Mrs. G came to my medical office she was quite worried, even skeptical... She said, "I don't think you can do much for me. "

I examined her and got her to talk. She was more or less depressed. She had been going from doctor to doctor without being able to rid herself of her pain on urination. There was no clinical indication of an organic disorder. For 3 or 4 sessions, she couldn't relax properly. She claimed to have no improvement. However, in rolling palpation, I observed a perceptible "improvement" that she finally recognises at the end of a month and a half (40 days).

This acceptance is very important because it signifies that the patient has broken with the feeling of despair which made her think there could be nothing done. All patients must go through this fundamental stage.

As a Practitioner, I watch out for this moment where the patient accepts to get better. Because from then on I know that a cure has been attained.

Real improvement and perceived improvement

Often rolling palpation shows a rapid "improvement" at the end of one or two sessions. But the perceived "improvement" by the patient can be deferred by a week, even two, and sometimes longer.

There is a neurological explanation for this. In effect, if we can make improvements in a local problem (segmental level), the cerebral zones in conflict for years by the disease will not reconstruct immediately in energy. It is necessary that "the local improvement" becomes older to permit a global disappearance of exhaustion.

In other words, the local conflict must be stabilized for a long time before the compromised cerebral areas can show some improvement.

Do not recreate the conditions of disease

Mrs. J is 35 years old. Her back was operated on 2 or 3 times. She felt an improvement, but pain persisted and prevented her from returning to work. I look at the radiographical films and it's an Eiffel Tower... there are metalworks everywhere!

On the global level one could say that the life of Mrs. J had not been easy. She lost her mother at 20 years old. She lived with her father and her brother who is a cerebromotor disabled person. Difficulties encountered at the birth of her second child was the triggering event for her low back pain.

She finally looked for a surgical solution for her problem. In intervening on a local level, surgery exacerbated problems that had been benign ones until then.

In reality, her main problem was not in her back. Her primary condition was that of exhaustion, a burn-out that had evolved into a state of frank depression. The pain was only the testimony of an unadapted organism that could no longer find an equilibrium. This is to say its capacity to take charge of difficulties, defeats, etc.

This is true for many patients who are caught up in a lesional view, which is true and valid in a way, but only represents 20 or 30 % of the reality of pain. When we operate on these patients, they get even more caught up and the result is catastrophic.

At the end of three or four sessions a young woman felt better. She admitted this and even spoke of a new awakening.

But she arrived for the fifth session very disappointed and said: "It's worse than ever! I can't take it anymore!"

"You don't even have to tell me. Because you felt better, so you could prove it to yourself, you recommenced all your previous activities and even more until the pain returned and finally you got exhausted again. Well, Madame, I can guarantee to you that you are really a thousand times better. But to affirm your new wellbeing you have recreated the disease which you resolved. Continue to live like that and you will never be cured."

Mr. D has back pain for 2 years. At the end of a month of treatment he is thinking about resuming his work as a carpenter. I try to dissuade him of this enthusiastic idea but without success. He relapses very quickly. When he is walking his dog he injures himself from a sudden somewhat forceful movement.

Like in the previous case, he had not yet been cured. In most cases of older diseases it takes several months.

Patients confuse the sense of happiness in feeling better with cure. And then spontaneously recreate the disease conditions as if they had completely forgotten about the past.

Clear the board of old problems

It's not because you lifted something heavy that you got injured. But the day you did, you should not have done it. It had become too difficult in regards to your rupture threshold. Your painful accident is the result of successive problems exceeding your adaptation capacity over time.

As long as you are stuck in old problems, you can no longer write on the blackboard of your life. Each time you write a word more, you run the risk of writing a word too much and to fall ill.

My role is to help you erase the board. I get rid of the old problems which weigh you down more and more and make you tired. If I can remove these old sufferings, I clean the board on which you are going to be able again to write.

Exactly as the therapist does on a psychological level I function on the neurological level.

Sports and neuromedicine: two "diabolical" disciplines

A sports activity is a brief moment of acceleration in life, a desired forceful activity defined in time. For our organism it is a momentaneous stress that is intercalated between long periods of rest. Like neuromedicine, a sports activity subjects the organism to lively stimulations that modify our behavior towards performing better. But it especially develops a resistance and allows for prevention of disease and early aging.

Moderate exercise is "atmospheric". It relaxes but does not result in disturbing the equilibrium.

An intense and prolonged exercise time can lead to a local rupture, favoring muscle pathologies for example. Unwise exercises create a durable exhaustion which can be severe. If on the one hand regular practice decreases incidence of cancer about 40 %, on the other hand, excessive practice can lead to a renewed outbreak of these diseases. Maximum benefit can be gained from short and dynamic workouts to obtain a neurologic response to stress. It is seen in the respiratory and cardiovascular impact and by the transpiration which occurs at 20 or 30 minutes after the beginning of the session. That is "turbo" exercise. The impact of sports favors resistance of the nervous system by raising up the rupture threshold for stress. It stimulates our basic functions: pain, inflammation, vascular tone, muscle tone and mood.

Numerous scientific works convince us of the interest of sports in the prevention of disease, such as cancer, cardiovascular diseases and degenerative neuronal diseases.

It affects our intellectual capacities too. Scrabble players or those who do crosswords think they do enough to maintain their brain. However, if they gave 10 % of their time of doing their favorite pastime to a brisk walk they would multiply by as much their competence to play both in performance and time played.

This neurologic aspect is little known in a discipline seemingly uniquely involving the body. Our Cartesian minds attribute to it a capacity to perform better physically and even to render more attractive our athletic body. In fact, its benefit is a global one which renders our nervous system just as effective as our body. "Washes your pen as it writes," says a famous advertisement. Likewise, sports maintain our neurons while muscles are at work!

At 50 years old, Mr. W, who works a lot, discovers he suffers from bilateral arthritis of the hips. On the occasion of a stressful workout, he felt a pain in both sides of his pelvis. This pain got worse to the point of disabling him. But he noticed that after 2 hours of walking it got better! Thanks to walking and one session of neuromedicine every three months, these pains decreased little by little over time, then disappeared.

Without the exercise, he would have been operated on much earlier. He had an operation 12 years after the appearance of the first pain.

Since then, he continues to exercise regularly, to consult a neuromedical doctor and has a busy professional life.

At least, walk!

I never saw anyone who started walking that did not get a benefit out of it in terms of performance and well-being. At the end of several weeks they feel less pain after exercise and they improve their performances. Only those who don't walk don't get any benefit. The latter say they are tired and have knee pains or back pains. In this renunciation, there is a counter truth. Walking, without regard to the intensity or the person walking, maintains specific functions and stimulates the organism. In practicing walking pain and fatigue will decrease in all of us, however, pleasure in it remains uncertain.

Other actions of stimulation

But I don't think that sport is the only factor leading to a better adaptation potential. Music, literature or spiritual development through brain stimulation acts specifically. It gives tonus, permits maybe maintaining a healthy equilibrium among persons, more so than those who are prisoners of their passion, ego, family conflicts or other conflicts.

What has preceded is to say that all actions that tend to stimulate the organism in a positive way, when reaching a certain threshold, are like a tool of neurofunctional re-education: effort, pain on effort and adaptation.

Disease to awaken health

Some patients are unfortunately confronted with severe diseases that affect their structural equilibrium.

Many more dramatise their condition and use it. They use it to justify behaviours that precisely contributed to make them ill. They withdraw in their symptomatology and difficultly accept any re-evaluation of their mode of life.

However, the "little" diseases should be a way to allow for an awakening of health: what did I not do to be in good health? Why have I fallen ill?

It is not a question of finding certain guilty parties or to look for scapegoats. Disease is a chance to reflect on what was too much done or not enough, on equilibriums that are upset. This is a unique chance to ask oneself about eating habits, relationships with others, the respect we owe ourselves and life as it has been given to us. And especially our health capital. How have we preserved this, managed this?

Disease is the point of arrival in an old life and the point of departure in renewal enriched by what we have learned through it.

15 Neurofunctional medicines

"The Trinity of Man body, spirit and neuroenergy."

The world of neurofunctional practices

Neuromedicine is not the only neurofunctional medicine. The medicines that I would like to join together are those aiming to stimulate the organism: acupuncture, thermal baths, massage, osteopathy, chiropractic medicine, etc.

Many of these techniques have existed for millenniums. So it is that man learned 3 or 4 000 years ago how to stimulate himself to perform better.

- Traditional Chinese Medicine (TCM) and Acupuncture

I feel very close to this global medicine. This technique also uses needles over what is called meridians. As we have seen already, these meridians are not the same as the dermatome circuits which are used in neuromedicine.

To break with my habitual treatment and renew my sensations I have treated patients with acupuncture needles. To vary the techniques allows for exploration of other possible responses.

The rolling palpation results are identical to that of neuromedicine. Even some times the relief seems deeper.

Nevertheless, it seems to me that TCM imposes a thought process that belongs to a different culture, on the patient. Neuromedicine is situated in this vein which puts back the patient in the center of the playing field. Nevertheless, it is to be seen as a part of Western Thinking. Without opposing what is modern, it hopes to link up with the roots of its culture. To reconcile man today in his global physical and cultural sense, which in the West is not Chinese...

- Thermal baths

There is not a fundamental difference between the principles of thermal baths and neuromedicine. In both cases, one acts on the unadapted patient and not on a specific disease. These two medicines also have in common the cutaneous neurological stimulations, whether we do it through thermal jets or with our little injections of magnesium.

In thermal baths, it is held that thermal water acts because it contains active agents. I am opposed to this restrictive conventional approach.

Whether in neuromedicine or thermal baths, treatment of chronic conditions at a given moment leads to a necessary critical point. While everything was seemingly better, the thermal bath patient suddenly feels pain and fatigue. The patient enters into a resistance stage: it is the thermal crisis that is going to allow restarting a deep and durable global response. This conception of reality escapes the doctors who are so divided in their theories, each one relieving pain of an organ in question. If in contrast to neuromedicine thermal baths don't treat acute conditions, they permit

patients to come out of their daily routine for a special beneficial period of care.

- Mesotherapy

We have already discussed at length this medicine practice
from which I derive. It purports to be a microdose conventional medicine. This positioning by mesotherapists permits them to remain in the confines of university medicine
and all the better.

But there is an error in this conception that prevents mesotherapy from taking the place it deserves in the functional
dimension of therapy.

In acute states, it possesses the same powers of neuromedicine. However, in chronic conditions, its treatment is limited by a conventional view and thus by the absence of a
global therapeutic approach of the patient which can only
be achieved by taking the time.

- Osteopathy and Chiropractic Medicine

Osteopaths and Chiropractors since 20 years ago are more
and more present in the life of patients. These disciplines
proved themselves efficient on bone relief, joint pain and
numerous other disease states such as digestive, sleep and
mood disorders, and stress.

Just like neuromedicine these methods of treatment can be considered transversal. It can intervene on numerous functions or diseased organs.

As a manual technique, it acts by a deep neuro-stimulation on tendons and fascias, while neuromedicine exercises in a first step cutaneous receptors.

It is rooted in a mechanical dimension. This medical term is an aberration for me but it's an image of pathology that patients can understand! It is derived from the treatment: displacement, putting back in place.

Osteopathy proves itself efficient in a context of a critical target organ and in acute cases more than in chronic ones, except for breakthrough pain in chronic diseases.

My deep personal conviction is that it has limited or no effect in severe diseases or older pathologies.

The advantages of osteopathy are multiple: efficiency, absence of toxicity, prevention. However, there is always a question about the validity of diagnoses given the nature of the medical training of osteopaths. It would be better if they were real doctors...

- Homeopathy

Homeopathy proves itself to be more efficient in functional diseases than in organic ones. For example, it relieves pain in arthritis and can prevent breakthroughs, but it can't reverse the evolution.

The prescription of infinitesimal doses acts in my opinion like internal stimulations. The intensity of the stimulations (dosage) is defined individually.

It shares with neuromedicine the distinction of a symptom and the global picture. Its action is in two phases: result in three days on the symptom and a global result in the patient at several months.

I would like to subject homeopathy to testing by rolling palpation. I would not be surprised to find similar results to those of cutaneous injections with a needle.

Moreover, this is just what is missing with homeopathy. The capacity to measure the outcome. For now, it can only rely on the subjective responses of its patients concerning its efficacy. In the case where the spontaneous outcome is often favorable, can it really claim to make a difference other than placebo effect?

- Medicinal plants or phytotherapy

Lots of drugs are made up of a base of plant extracts. We can consider this a branch of conventional medicine in a positive and natural light concerning the drug. Furthermore, certain plants have disgusting qualities that cause reactions similar to neurofunctional stimulations. For instance, the ancients purged themselves before winter by eating black radishes.

In the face of this ambiguity, herb doctors must be situated: are they conventional doctors using plants or are they re-educational therapists?

- Psychotherapy

Psychotherapy cannot be considered as a global medicine. Nevertheless, this discipline has, through its actions on mental health a real complementary effect to other "body medicines".

In fact, it operates by its applications to the feeling of the pain to create a reaction that can lead to the patient's escape from his rut. Psychotherapy provokes "microtraumas" when dealing with painful periods of the patient's life. In doing so, it gradually desensitizes the patient. It is the same principle in neuromedicine: it doesn't involve the needles, but an "aggressive" act as in all re-education.

In this way, it is a neurofunctional discipline.

- Popular Medicines

One can cite here the bonesetters, the magnetisers, Grandma's remedies and other ways to a cure that classical medicine prefers to ignore.

In a way, all of these medicines use the neurofunctional principle of stimulation. So they must not be rejected. They offer a treatment that plays down the disease and offers reassurance. They can prove to have great efficacy in disorders where a vital risk is not incurred.

In one of her books, my fellow doctor, Janine Fontaine explains that medicine men in the Philippines are not afraid to tackle any kind of disorder. Their goal is not so much to stop patients from dying but to give them time by rendering the organism the most able as possible to live in harmony with its pathology.

In the world of these neurofunctional practices, we have only discussed those that are most similar to neuromedicine. There should be a clearer distinction between practitioners of these disciplines: those who are doctors and those who are not, those who have a scientific background and those who do not, and those who intervene in the framework of popular empirical medicines.

But I don't want to exclude anyone, the world is so rich! We are wrong to ignore and often to combat them. It isn't bad that these practices are competing with modern medicine. The interesting thing is the synthesis we can make: a chance for the medicine of tomorrow...

- A guiding diagram

One can appreciate the fact that the world of neurologic re-education is immense but misunderstood. Since it is not organised it is seen as being too diverse.

I do not want for each medicine or each therapist to lose their specificity. In my view, the techniques aren't very important, what counts is the therapist on condition that he is aware of the limits and scope of his practice.

What I would like to see is that we stop going out to the public in disarray, and especially in front of health organisations who decide our future by misjudging our capacity to cure people.

I would like to see all these therapists recognise each others' capacities and to unite behind the idea of neurologic re-education in an associative framework. This would create a common thinking base for all neurofunctional medicines.

Each patient would be able to enter into a precise system of medical analysis whose criteria would have been defined.

The relationship with the neurosciences

Neurofunctional medicines are directly concerned by the development of the neurosciences because we act on the nervous system.

Neurosciences ignore us because they work "from the top". They are trying to define an anatomical and neurophysiological map of the nervous system. They are involved in the discovery and analysis of the brain, of the spinal cord and their impact on the functioning of the individual and his organs. In order to understand pain phenomena for instance, what are the involved zones? They identify the first, second zones, acceleration zones, and the zones that involve memory...

They focus on structures that are involved and more precisely on the neurohormones that are found in them. They are fundamentalists, whereas we are behaviourists with our practice of patients.

Neuroscience explains the diagrams I have shown here. In a reciprocal way, I should think that our approach should lead the way to fundamental research by offering neuro-science a concrete entry into general medical practice.

Neuromedicine sees man in three ways: the body, the spirit, and thirdly the neurofunctional threshold. In a fundamental way, neurosciences should be interested in this third sector. Humanity needs this investigation to better understand how diseases are cured by neuromedicine.

I am thinking about all chronic or allergic diseases.

Such as cystic fibrosis. I know how to help these patients gain 5 to 10 years of comfort by trying to eliminate the major part of the neurologic medullary and spinal cord suffering caused by their disease. I am also thinking of other pathologies such as myocardiopathies. In my opinion, these are secondary, uniquely neurologic diseases after cardiac suffering. We find them after a myocardial infarct or IHD (Ischemic Heart Disease).

I am thinking of scoliosis, which has finally been recognized as a neurologic functional disease and not a vertebral one. The same is true for kyphosis.

I am also thinking of all the immobilised patients in a hospital bed who could use dynamic re-education to reduce the risk of occurrence of a chronic condition as best as is possible.

I don't doubt that neurofunctional medicines will finally be recognised and find their defined place in medicine, especially in prevention, treatment of pain and fatigue.

Conclusion

"We know that nature always has the upper hand. While waiting until that day when she totally dominates us, we can divert. some of her force to our own ends."

This is a delicate position in which I am presenting myself. Am I a doctor one among so many fellow doctors? Am I a Guru?

Yes, I assume the responsibility of being different than my fellow doctors. I am more interested in patients than diseases. But no, I do not pretend to hold a revelation of truth.

Am I a revolutionary?

No, an observer, a doctor engaged in a unique adventure for patients and a return to an equilibrium for disease. I do not consider myself to be original, just to be desirous of constructing a true way of thinking. I have gone further than merely the results called for in the "criteria for good medical practice". I like to understand so as not to submit to fate.

Am I a savant at the top of his game?

Yes, I created a medicine of it's time based on empiric results, which have been analysed, making it a scientific endeavor. A medicine beginning to take shape.

I am alone still, but I would like to establish a school of my own...

This book is written for my patients but also is a call to my fellow doctors to convince them that the time has come to think about medicine in a different way. Diseases have evolved. In 1900, 30% of the French population had syphilis and even more suffered from tuberculosis. Medicine was confronted with daily survival scenarios. It had to find radical solutions at the scale of whole populations.

Thanks to medicine, Western patients can finally profit from their protected body. But today, this medicine has lost its face against emerging diseases, consequences of rapid modifications of the environment and lifestyle.

The time of the grandiose medical conquests where the tragedy of the situations called for big means should give way to a more detailed approach that is more focused on the future of a patient. More than ever, patients should take responsibility for their health and diseases.

Medicine heavily intervenes in all pathologies under the fallacious pretext that the risk must not be taken. Disastrous error. This requirement for an immediate efficacy which is rarely needed at first makes the patient go astray from possible knowledge of his disease and himself. Here, our organs seem to have more value than ourselves. Such an attitude takes the credibility of doctors away. It undermines their diagnostic prowess and their "outlook". It confuses all conditions in a real or potential severity in prescribing tests, exams, or treatments and it legitimizes itself rather than actually reaching a cure. It does not support the patient in finding their way but encourages them to consume drugs, which shut them up into a standardization of their condition and their aspirations for good health.

I apologise to those who are offended. I am a general practitioner. See only in these few words a defense, voluntarily biased, for the survival of this medicine. It is responsible for the global quality of daily life, of the future of each patient, but also the future of everyone searching for good health. It has criteria based on proof (Evidence Based Medicine) and it is far from any play-acting. The acute conditions and severe diseases are rare in general practice. It is more orientated around the patient than the disease. The latter remains the responsibility of the organic specialists who, despite their empathy, cannot make a triage of minor problems that hobble us.

It is generally agreed that we are advancing into an era of more and more invasive and sophisticated specialization when medical research should orient itself towards prevention and treatment of neurologic diseases of exhaustion. These will affect 100% of the population and will be the subject of tomorrow's medicine. Many neglected conditions in our time present a predictive and preventive dimension that is taken into account by a patient-orientated medicine. The growing role of alternative medicines forces us to reflect on the patient's world. The patient is demanding new requirements. Are patients escaping from a "medical care factory" that frightens them or are they running after the panacea of complementary medical measures? Whatever the reason, they are looking for alternatives. They are looking for a treatment closer to them and, in their eyes, more efficient.

Neuromedicine is tinged by this new approach, and at the same time being an efficient technique. My results are proof of this. My patients believe in it. To them, the goal is not to get better in episodes but to have a long-lasting cure. With or without associated treatment, neuromedicine permits treatment of the diverse components of their condition, leading to a stable equilibrium that protects them.

I believe that a medicine without philosophy, without a humanist agenda, cannot be a medicine. It is a technical act, a materialist medicine and by consequence a one-off medicine with no sense of time. Relieving a passive ailment, it ignores the future. Patients rebuild themselves out of the fear of a relapse, not in the finality of the hope of a new life. Neuromedicine confers a philosophical dimension to its action. As it appropriates times, neuromedicine carries two hopes: improving the future of individual patients by helping them conceive of a painless tomorrow; contributing to a collective betterment for a more conscious and confident society.

Feeling sure about this certain truth, I am open to other re-educational neurofunctional medicines. And I dream of ending the controversy with conventional medicine in order to find a common ground upon which today we can begin to work together.

Treat Life with Life!

Glossary

A

Acute

This is a term used to describe a disease or inflammation that is active for a brief time.

Adaptation

The capacity to react to a stimulus in such a way as to ensure homeostasis or energy equilibrium.

Addiction

The physical or psychological dependence on a drug or activity.

Aging

The natural physiological process of getting older.

Alzheimer's Disease

A degenerative debilitating disease causing dementia.

Arc Reflex

Spinal response to a cutaneous stimulus which results in an automatic movement [Diagram].

Autonomic Nervous System

An automatic inherent nervous system in the body that ensures life without respect to any voluntary actions. It is divided into the Sympathetic Nervous System and the Parasympathetic Nervous System which act in opposite ways but both act in order to ensure homeostasis.

B

Bagot, René (1908-1981)

Rheumatologist. In 1952 he recreated and led a thalassotherapy center in Roscoff, Brittany founded in 1899 by his father Louis Bagot. He was pioneer in the development of the rolling palpation technique used in treatment, diagnosis and follow-up of neuromedicine.

Bellestros, Daniel

A contemporary French doctor who developed body energy theory using Kirlian Effect of recording body energy on a photographic plate on the foot of patients and an early mesotherapist and homeopathist.

Balneotherapy

Hydrotherapy with sea water or hot springs water. There are thalassotherapy stations and hot spas in many parts of France.

Bernard, Claude (1813-1878)

A famous French 19th Century pioneer doctor and great scientist. Modern medicine owes this researcher alot. He was a proponent of the experimental method, which he described in his main work Introduction to Experimental Medicine.

Burn Out

A psychiatric and physical condition characterised by an extreme exhaustion due to previous psychological and physical overloads by stresses encountered at work.

C

Cancer

A multitude of diseases caused by a mutation in one cell of the body which multiplies and causes damage to other cells and organs.

Cartography

The cutaneous representation of deep sensibility of various organs according to maps proposed by three original doctors: H. Head of England (1861-1960), Jules Déjerine (1849-1817) and H. Jarricot in France. This cartography follows precise representations in the dermatomes. It is a common basis for many treatments like in osteopathy, acupuncture, neuromedicine and reflexology. One can no doubt add thalassotherapy and thermal baths.

Chiropractor

A doctor trained in manipulation of the body in order to correct blockages.

Chronic

As opposed to acute this term indicates a long-term disorder 3 months to many years in progress often occuring at
older age (but not necessarily).

Complementary Medicine

As opposed to Conventional Medicine this englobes the
alternative medical sciences used in such disciplines as homeopathy, acupuncture, osteopathy, botanical medicine,
and neuromedicine. It does not involve prescribing chemical drugs or surgical procedures.

Conventional Medicine

The current scientific practice of using chemical prescription drugs for disease or using surgical procedures in organic lesions as proved by evidence-based medicine.

D

Dermatomes

Areas on the skin stemming from embryological tissues
which correspond to a specific nerve function.

Diclofenac

An effective non-steroidal antinflammatory drug sometimes used in very small diluted doses for the microinjections of mesotherapy.

E

Energetic Potential

The amount of energy in reserve that can be used to face
new physical or psychological conflicts or stresses which
allows adaptation to occur.

Evidence-Based Medicine

The scientific analytical and Tquantitative approach to
medical problems based on definitive evidence of any particular pathology or lesion.

It is used to evaluate efficacy. As discovery of actions of
lemons and oranges for treatment of scurvy.

Exhaustion

The mental and physical state or condition of a patient
which arises when the energy reserves are expended in the
long term and a deficit in body balance occurs. It may be
the result of reiterated stressful conditions that form a defined neurological state.

F

Fibromyalgia

A newly-described controversial disease characterised by chronic severe pains in the muscles and causing disability.

G

Galen (129-216AD)

A 2nd Century AD philosopher and doctor of Greek origin born in Bergamon working in Rome who revamped and systematized the theories of Hippocrates. His works were followed until the Renaissance by medieval doctors. He described the four humours and vital spirit.

Grandma's Remedies

Naturopathic or botanical remedies handed down in families generation after generation for treatment of illnesses based on an empirical and subjective experience in their use.

H

Hippocrates (460-370BC)

The Founder of Scientific Medicine who worked on the Greek Island of Cos. He formed

a body of medicinal information based on logic and not magic or religion. Illness was considered as a natural phenomenon. Today doctors worldwide take the Hippocratic Oath on graduation from medical school.

Holistic Medicine

An approach to medical science which takes into account both the body and spirit. In neuromedicine this includes neuroenergy and the physical and psychological equilibrium of each patient.

Homeopathy

A medical approach discovered by a German doctor Samuel Hahneman (1755-1843) based on treatment using infinitessimal dilutions of active preparations.

Homeostasis

The continuous process of the body and its organs to maintain a steady state of equilibrium allowing for maximal organ functions and avoiding any failures.

Hypothalamus

Big as an almond it is located at the base of the brain under the cortex. It is comprised of numerous nuclei and manages the autonomic nervous system. Numerous behaviours are regulated including hunger, thermoregulation and sexuality through neurohormones which are secreted. It stimulates the

secretion of other neurohormones by the pituitary gland and endocrine organs. It is a relay between neurobiological reality and endocrine functions.

I

Immunity

The body's defences against foreign substances or germs divided into cellular immunity (white blood cells) and humoral immunity (antibodies).

Infection

A disease state caused by microorganisms like viruses, bacteria, mycobacteria, fungi or parasites (malaria by sporozoa) and is often characeised by swelling, redness, warmth and pain with pus formation. It is very often accompanied by a fever and organ failure if severe.

Inflammation

A local disease state caused by a tissular disorder including redness, swelling, warmth but no puand pain in which macrophages cells are abundant and other white blood cells and many humoral factors such as interleukins and prostaglandins It may occur spontaneously or be the result of an injury. Neuromedicine corrects especially the prolonged inflammatory state in chronic diseases but also in acute disorders.

L

Leriche, René(1879-1955)

Surgeon and French physiologist. He was recruited in WWI and worked

in pain and vascular surgery. He departed with the strictly organic view of pathology and was interested in the role of the nervous system.

Like Claude Bernard, he proposed a functional theory of sickness through the role of the sympathetic nervous system. He fought for a human based surgery and said: "The pain relief issue leads to a human-based medicine in all its forms".

Lesion

A deleterious change in deep or superficial tissues caused by either traumatic injury or disease.

Lidocaïne

An anaesthetic sometimes used in small diluted doses in the microinjections of mesotherapeutic and neuromedical treatment.

M

Magnesium

The 12th element in Mendeleev's Chart, an alkaline metal with two positive charges, is important in the functions of the nerves, the muscles and the heart. It is well-known for its anti-stress characteristics and is widely used in neuro-medicine in the dilutions of subcutaneous microinjections.

Meridians

These are the virtual lines on the body used in Acupuncture to locate an appropriate point for the use of the acupuncture needle in the presence of a particular pathology. Pain elicited in rolling palpation permits validating meridians. The needle of acupuncture relieves the pain in about 10 minutes.

Mesotherapy

A microdosed conventional medical approach for treatment of pain and diseases involving multiple or single microinjections of various drugs into the subcutaneous tissues. Cf. Michel Pistor It is also used in cosmetic medicine for cellulitis and wrinkles.

Microinjections

Subcutaneous needle injections of a very small quantity of active product used in neuromedicine and mesotherapy.

Mréjen, Didier

A doctor that developed Punctual Systematised Mesotherapy, an acupuncture-like technique where drugs are injected in specific points of the back at a given distance from the spine.

Muscle Tone

The steady-state level of muscle contractions which is permanent even when at rest.

N

Nerve Plexus

A mass of nervous tissue that conducts specific functional activities in the body.

Nervous System

The network of nerves in the body, spîne and brain.

Neuroenergy

The vital force that animates the body which permits neurological adaptation.

Neurofunctional Reeducation

Used by all the complementary medical disciplines. It considers that the nervous system is in the center of the disease process. It is a cure for specific states.

Neurogenic pain

Arising from sensitive nerves when no evidence of an organic lesion is found such as in patients with algodystrophy or phantom pains in amputees. This type of pain is often very severe and chronic and responds well to neuromedical treatment.

Nocebo

The negative effect felt by patients when a treatment has been carried out which may result in a positive result later as seen in the 3-day evolution of a neuromedical treatment.

O

Obesity

A state of overweightedness characterised by a Body Mass Index of over 30.

Organ

A functional tissular unit in the body that has some autonomy and is most often essential to life.

Osteopathy

The medical practice developed in 1870 by Andrew Taylor Still in Kansas, USA based on anatomical realities that involves manipulations to deblock injured or inflamed body parts. It is often used in sports medicine.

P

Pain

A nervous sensation in the brain with specific nervous pathways in the body. Pain is often the result of a disease process. It may be acute or chronic.

Paré, Ambroise(1510-1590)

Surgeon and French anatomist. Often considered as the father

of modern surgery, he invented many instruments. At the battleside he learned to put ligatures on vessels to cauterize wounds renouncing the common practice of using boiling oil as violent. Surgeon and Barber in his early career – who didn't speak either Latin or Greek in spite of

the University, he finished by being official surgeon of French Kings Henri II to Henri IV. He wrote several medical books.

Phytotherapy

The medicinal science of botanical medicine.

Pistor, Michel(1924-2003)

French doctor who founded mesotherapy.

Placebo

A drug preparation containing no active principles. It is used to evaluate the real effect of drugs.

Placebo Effect

State of a patient feeling better after any treatment specific or not. It is a psychological or neurological effect.

Popular Medicine

The group of medical approaches which are used based on an empirical and subjective groundwork not generally approved by the Conventional Evidence-Based Medical Community.

Postcure

That period of time following treatment such as in cancer with chemotherapy, radiotherapy or surgery that is characterised by a number of side effects. It responds well to neuromedical treatment.

Prevention

It acts before onset of disease. The rolling palpation technique allows the practitioner to detect infraclinical or asymptomatic lesional or inflammatory conditions in the body and then treat them. Thus the symptomatic form of disease is avoided.

R

Readaptation

The resulting state after cure that permits a global both organic and psychological rehabilitation.

Reconstruction

The global rebuilding of energy stores once these have been exhausted.

Resolution

The finding of a solution once an exhaustion has occurred.

Rolling Palpation

The technique used to diagnose and for follow-up verification of efficacy. It involves a rolling and pinching of the skin over the dermatomes and plexus cartography of the body. It can be used for cure as well as in a thalassotherapy center due to its stimulative effect over the cutaneous tissues.

S

Segmentary

Peripheral level of nervous activity and pain which is spinal not involving the brain centers.

Sideration

The general state of semi-euphoria occurring after any positive or negative trauma. In neuromedicine it immediately follows stimulation by microinjections.

Sports

Leisure activities which require physical exercise of the body. It is a strong stimulation of the body which modifies in time physical and/ or psychological behaviour. It has a protective effect on the body.

Stimulation

Activation of a nervous impulse in the body which results in an effect having a beneficial impact on the body and spirit.

Suprasegmentary

The level of nervous activity which is central like in the brain beginning where the spinal cord leaves off in the neck.

T

Thalamus

A bilateral organ located between the cerebral cortex and the medulla oblongata. Its two parts are separated by the third ventricle. All the sensory and sensible nerves of the body go through it and it modulates perception by activation or inhibition. It intervenes also in motor function and consciousness. It activates vigilance in diurnal phase and induces sleep in nocturnal phase (slow sleep). It is composed of numerous nucleii for multiple afferents and efferents especially cortical and cerebellar ones.

Threshold

The point of negative stimulation which causes pain to appear or of positive stimulation which causes pain to disappear.

Traditional Chinese Medicine

An approach to medical treatment which is based on 3 millenia of practice using botanical medicines and/or acupuncture.

Triggering Event

A life event which often corresponds with the appearance of a pathological painful condition.

Tunnel, The

an underground passage. The phase of the healing process in neuromedical treatment characterised by a slow-going improvement and rather important feeling of discouragement on the part of the patient. It may occur in neuromedical treatment of chronic pain between the 2nd and 4th weeks of treatment.

Turbo

The neurological acceleration of the healing process.

This book was written based on an abundant number of French references by such notable authors as Antonio Damasio, Daniel Ballestros, Didier Mrejen, etc.

Table of Contents

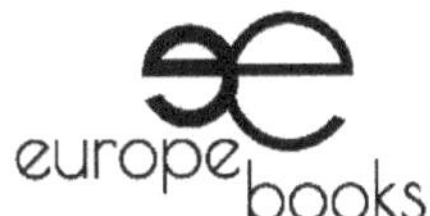